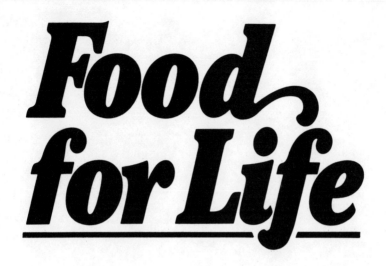

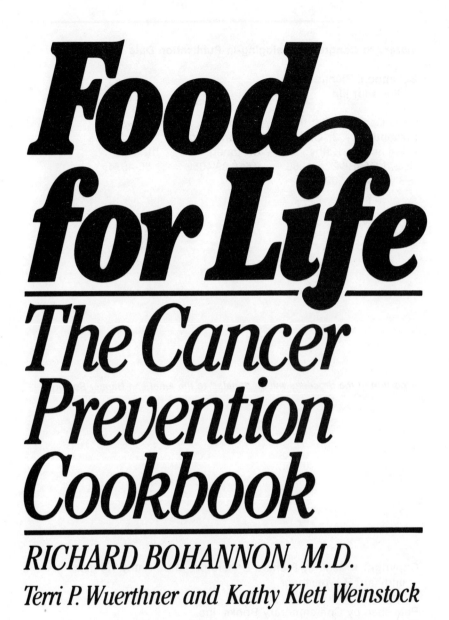

Food for Life

The Cancer Prevention Cookbook

RICHARD BOHANNON, M.D.

Terri P. Wuerthner and Kathy Klett Weinstock

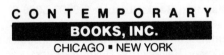

CONTEMPORARY
BOOKS, INC.
CHICAGO ▪ NEW YORK

Library of Congress Cataloging-in-Publication Data

Bohannon, Richard.
  Food for life.

  1. Cancer—Diet therapy—Recipes.   2. Cancer—
Prevention.   3. Cancer—Nutritional aspects.
I. Weinstock, Kathy.   II. Wuerthner, Terri.   III. Title.
RC271.D52B64   1986   616.99′4052   86-4574
ISBN 0-8092-5029-2

A portion of the proceeds will be donated to the American Cancer Society.

Published by Contemporary Books, Inc.
180 North Michigan Avenue, Chicago, Illinois 60601
Manufactured in the United States of America
Library of Congress Catalog Card Number: 86-4574
International Standard Book Number: 0-8092-5029-2

Published simultaneously in Canada by Beaverbooks, Ltd.
195 Allstate Parkway, Valleywood Business Park
Markham, Ontario L3R 4T8 Canada

This book is dedicated with much love to Margaret E. Klett

Contents

Contents

Acknowledgments

The authors would like to thank all the many people who worked so long and hard on this book, especially our nutritionist, Elaine Moquette, R.D., for her relentless dedication to perfection in her part of the work; our agents, Joyce Cole and Jayne Walker, for their confidence and patience, with special thanks to Jayne for her invaluable editorial assistance; Helen Jones, Director of Communications, American Cancer Society, San Francisco Chapter, for her encouragement and help with the project; and to Bonnie Willacker for her time, which she gave so willingly.

Very loving thanks go to our spouses, Nancy Bohannon, Dick Wuerthner, and Jordan Weinstock, for tasting countless recipes and for helping whenever and wherever needed as our involvement in the book consumed almost all our time. Without the love, support, and encouragement of these three people, this book never would have been possible.

Our wonderful kids—Robert Bohannon; Michele, Dawn, and Diana Wuerthner; and Andrea, Barry, Daniel, and Peter Weinstock—deserve an award for their patience during the last three years. Without our families, there would have been little reason to write a book such as this. It truly was a labor of love.

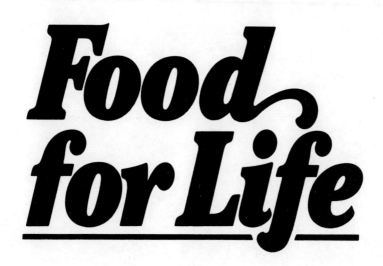

Introduction

"... The weight of evidence suggests that what we eat during our lifetime strongly influences the probability of developing certain cancers. ..."

—from *Diet, Nutrition, and Cancer*, published in 1982 by the National Research Council

This quiet statement has set off a storm in the four years since its release. Articles, essays, and books have poured from the media in a steady stream, echoing and reverberating this message.

Why? Because for the first time, a careful appraisal of published studies clearly indicates that *how we eat* can have an impact on whether or not we develop cancer. That in fact, by best estimates, 35% of all human cancers are *diet-related*.

The impact of this news is riveting: We *can* have some control over this dreaded disease, starting in our own kitchens.

But there is also some confusion surrounding the diet/cancer connection. We are aware that changing to a certain diet may prevent cancer, but we aren't sure what changes to make. In my medical practice, my patients ask many questions about this connection: "Will eating a lot of carrots every day prevent lung cancer?" "Should I take megadoses of vitamin C to prevent (or cure) cancer?" "Is it true that if I follow a diet of brown rice and vegetables I won't ever get cancer?" Even though the direct answer to all of these questions is no, there is a kernel of truth in all of them:

1

- Carrots are high in beta-carotene, which converts to vitamin A in the body. When eaten in liberal doses, carrots and other beta-carotene rich vegetables have been shown in some studies to prevent cancers of the lung and bladder.
- There are also benefits to eating an abundance of vitamin-C-rich fruits and vegetables. In some cases, they have been shown to reduce the incidence of cancer of the esophagus and stomach.
- And a diet of brown rice and vegetables, if balanced correctly, is a wonderful low-fat, high-fiber diet, which has been associated with a low incidence of cancer in general.

What my coauthors and I have done in this book is to condense all the scientific information on diet and its role in cancer prevention into a practical and flavorful way of eating to reduce the risk of cancer. Although research on the diet/cancer connection is still in its early stages, the connection is clearly there. We have used the *Interim Guidelines* of the National Research Council, and the nutrition guidelines of the American Cancer Society, in preparing the text and recipes in this book.

These guidelines suggest the following:

- reduce the amount of fat in your diet
- eat more fresh fruits, vegetables, and whole grains
- minimize your consumption of smoked or salt-cured foods
- drink alcohol only in moderation.

If these guidelines sound simple, it is because they are. Better still, they aren't suggesting drastic or unattainable diet changes, but rather a *redirection* of your way of eating: You should simply eat *more* of some foods and *less* of others.

But which foods are good and which are bad? Let's look a little more closely at the guidelines.

STEP 1: REDUCE FAT INTAKE

This is the most important step on a cancer risk–reduction diet.

There is no way around it. We *must* cut down on our present intake of fat. We eat far too many foods on a regular basis that are high in fat. Statistics show that an average of 40% of our total calories a day come from fat. The *Interim Guidelines* recommend that we limit our fat intake to no more than 30% of total calories per day. This means that the average American has to cut his or her fat intake by one fourth.

More than any other dietary consideration, fat has been linked to high cancer rates of the breast, colon, gall bladder, ovaries, uterus, and prostate. This is why we should be eating less fat than we do now—not a difficult task if you follow a few simple rules.

1. Starting in the supermarket, always buy the leanest cuts of meat. Then before cooking, trim off any visible fat. If you cook lean cuts of meat properly, they will be flavorful and tender.

2. Buy chicken and fish more often than you buy red meat. Remove the skin from poultry, and you remove a big portion of the fat.

3. Start serving smaller portions of meat, fish, or poultry, and bigger portions of vegetables. We Americans take pride in the portion sizes that we serve. Think of all the restaurants that boast the *thickest steak* or the *biggest slab of prime rib* in town. Rather than keeping us healthy, these gargantuan portions may be taking years off our lives. The amount of fat in 12 or 16 ounces of red meat is staggering. The average adult needs, at most, only 3 or 4 ounces of meat, fish, or poultry at a meal in order to have a healthy diet.

Compare our American diet to the typical Japanese diet. You will notice that they eat more fish, rice, and vegetables than meat. It is interesting to note that when Japanese women move to our country and adopt our high-fat, meat-oriented diet, their rate of breast cancer increases substantially. Japanese women living in Japan ordinarily have a very low rate of breast cancer.

4. Cook with little or no fat. The way you cook affects the amount of fat in your diet. Every time you fry food you greatly increase the amount of fat in the meal. Admittedly, fried foods may taste good, but that's the fat you are tasting, not the food. It is possible to cook with little or no fat by cooking instead with wine, herbs, and juices (lemon juice for example). They not only flavor the food but moisten it as well. Many of our chapter introductions include a "Cooking Methods" section that shows you how to cook a variety of foods using little or no fat.

5. Eat meatless meals at least once or twice a week. Animal protein from meats like beef and pork can contain up to 75% of their calories from fat, while the staples of vegetarian meals— beans, rice, lentils, peas, and other legumes—contain only 5 to 15% of their calories from fat. For those of you with little experience with vegetarian meals, you have a treat in store—

they can be absolutely delicious. One of the most famous and elegant restaurants here in San Francisco, Greens, is vegetarian. It is so popular that reservations have to be made weeks in advance.

Chapter 5, Meatless Entrées, offers some exciting dishes that will please vegetarians, and, we hope, intrigue those of you who are cooking meatless meals for the first time. Researchers have studied with great interest the cancer rates of a vegetarian religious group in our country, the Seventh Day Adventists. They eat no animal protein; the staples of their diets are fruits, vegetables, and whole grains. Their overall cancer rate is extremely low compared to that of other groups. Another study done in England and Wales during a 50-year period from 1928 to 1978 showed that during World War II, as the fat consumption went down because of the shortage of meat, eggs, and butter, and as the staples of the diet became vegetables and whole grains, the breast cancer rate dropped significantly. It shot up again in the postwar years when these foods became easily available again. Cancer of the breast has been linked to high intakes of fat in many other population studies.

Another reason to reduce dietary fat is to reduce the likelihood of becoming overweight. Studies done by the American Cancer Society show that people who are considered obese (and especially those weighing at least 40% more than average body weight) have an overall higher rate for many common cancers including breast, colon, uterine, and prostate than those people who are in the normal to slightly under normal weight range. Fat, here again, is the culprit.

6. Make sure every meal and snack you eat *contains no more than 30% calories from fat.* This means if your dinner entrée contains 35% calories from fat, your vegetable 10%, and your fruit 5%, chances are your total meal contains less than 30% calories from fat. See Chapter 10, 21-Day Menu Plan, for examples of what a 30%-calories-from-fat meal looks like.

Each of the recipes in this book has been computer-analyzed for several nutrients. The percentage of calories from fat is listed for each recipe.

But how do you calculate calories from fat when you are not using one of these recipes? Most food products will have the grams of fat per serving listed on the food label, along with the calories per serving. Take the grams of fat per serving, multiply by 9 (9 calories per gram of fat), divide this number by the number of calories per serving, and there you have it—the percentage of calories from fat.

For example, there are 5 grams of fat per serving of low-fat milk (2% milk fat) and 120 calories per one-cup serving: 5×9 (calories per gram) = 45 calories from fat; $45 \div 120$ (total calories per serving) = 37.5% calories from fat.

Obviously, foods like fresh broccoli, apples, or cantaloupe don't have an ingredient label. That's too bad; it would be a great way to advertise their health value. Look up these foods in Appendix II to figure grams of fat per serving and total calories per serving, calculating percentage of calories from fat as you did above. (Appendix II will also give the vitamin and fiber content of these foods.)

Meal Planning—How Much Fat?

Think about your usual breakfast. Do you eat a croissant or a donut on the run, or do you sit down to a bowl of whole-grain cereal with fruit and a glass of nonfat milk? The second breakfast adds up to no more than 30% calories from fat. But be careful—some breakfast cereals (including many granola varieties) by themselves contain around 40% calories from fat: check the label. If you like toast in the morning, add up your toast, what you put on it, exactly how much you eat, and whatever else you eat or drink. Then total it up. Make substitutions and decrease quantities from fat sources until the meal adds up to no more than 30% calories from fat.

For lunch, bag it with foods you know are within the guidelines, using leftover dinner entrées from recipes in this book and reheating them up at work or at home. Or take vegetable sticks, a slice of low-fat cheese like part-skim mozzarella, whole-wheat crackers or bread, and a piece of fruit.

For dinner, use any of the seafood, poultry, meat, or meatless entrée recipes in this book, until you feel you know what a low-fat entrée is; then you can start creating your own, making substitutions and following the general cooking guidelines described in the chapter sections. Besides the entrée chapters, we have a marvelous Sauces and Salad Dressings chapter. Some of these low-fat sauces can dress up plain chicken or fish so deliciously that you wouldn't guess you are eating a meal low in fat.

Try to plan each meal so that *each* is 30% calories from fat. For example, don't eat a no-fat breakfast and then eat a 60%-calories-from-fat lunch. The whole idea of a cancer risk–reduction diet is to *balance* fats, fiber, and vitamins at every meal.

STEP 2: INCREASE INTAKE OF FRESH FRUITS, VEGETABLES, AND WHOLE GRAINS

We'd like to stress again that people whose diets regularly include fresh fruits, vegetables, and whole grains have low cancer rates. The common denominator of fruits, vegetables, and whole grains—why they are so good for you—is that they all contain good amounts of dietary fiber, and many contain good amounts of vitamins A and C.

The Fiber Connection

The role of fiber in reducing the risk of cancer needs to be made clearer. Dietary fiber includes several nondigestible food elements. When these elements go through the intestines, they shorten the time that other food elements are in the gastrointestinal tract. Current thought is that the shorter the time any harmful elements are in the body, the less time they will have to do any damage.

The average American diet is considered very low in fiber—about 10 grams a day. The National Cancer Institute recommends 25 to 35 grams of fiber per day—a goal that is easy to attain if you eat the right amount of the foods that are high in fiber. You don't need to consume great amounts of unprocessed bran, cereals full of wood pulp, or equally unsavory things to get this amount of fiber. By eating a liberal amount of fruits, vegetables (including beans and peas), and whole grains—whole-wheat breads and cereals, natural rice, rolled oat cereals, and cornmeal products—you can easily get the required amounts of fiber. Populations with diets high in fiber have less cancer of the colon and breast than do those people who eat low-fiber diets. If people only ate enough dietary fiber, they wouldn't be plagued with constipation and have to resort to laxatives to keep their systems "regular."

High-Fiber Foods

Refer to the nutritional chart in Appendix II for foods and their fiber contents and see how many of your favorite foods—including snack foods like popcorn, fresh fruit, and sunflower seeds—contain this necessary food element. I am surprised at the number of my patients who have never tasted delicious whole foods like polenta, bulgur wheat, and whole-wheat pasta. Other good examples of high-fiber foods are corn and whole-wheat tortillas, blackberries, cantaloupe, lentils, wheat crackers, peas and beans, and oatmeal cookies—it's a surprisingly varied selection.

Refer to the fiber listings in Appendix II to make sure you are consuming between 25 and 35 grams of fiber per day. In general, begin choosing a variety of fruits (melons, apricots, grapefruit, oranges, peaches), a variety of vegetables (carrots, broccoli, cauliflower, potatoes, squash, greens), unfiltered fruit and vegetable juices, whole-grain breakfast cereals (oatmeal, shredded wheat), whole-wheat bread and bread products (whole-grain pasta, crackers), brown rice, dried beans and peas, seeds, popcorn, and nuts in moderate amounts (they are high in fat).

To ensure that the whole-wheat product you are about to buy is indeed made from whole-wheat flour, check the first ingredient on the label. It should say *whole-wheat flour. Cracked-wheat* or *wheat* products are usually made with enriched wheat flour (white flour), which contains practically no fiber per serving. Stay away from refined food products to ensure that you are getting the good fiber content whole food supplies in its natural state.

The Vitamin Connection

Along with dietary fiber, fruits and vegetables contain vitamins and other elements that have been shown to reduce the risk of cancer—namely *vitamin C, beta-carotene* (which converts to vitamin A), and *indoles* (found in cruciferous vegetables—those in the cabbage family).

- Vitamin C is difficult to talk about without recalling all that's been written about its healing effects—from the common cold to burns to cancer. We don't know if large doses of vitamin C will cure anything—but in some studies a *diet* high in vitamin C has been shown to reduce the occurence of cancers of the stomach and esophagus. Vitamin-C-rich fruits and vegetables include citrus fruits, strawberries, cantaloupe and other melons, broccoli, cabbage, green peppers, and most dark green leafy vegetables. Eating a luscious bowl of strawberries, a broccoli quiche, or some roasted green peppers is a satisfying alternative to consuming vitamin C in tablet form.
- Beta-carotene (vitamin A) is found in carrots, sweet potatoes, winter squash, apricots, peaches, cantaloupe,

and most dark green leafy vegetables. A general way to judge how much beta-carotene is contained in a fruit or vegetable is the deepness of the color. The more yellow-orange the food is or the darker the leaf of a vegetable, the more beta-carotene it contains. One really deep orange-colored vegetable is the sweet potato. One baked sweet potato contains 24,877 IU of vitamin A. If you serve this only once a year on Thanksgiving, you are missing the opportunity to get a good amount of this vitamin on a regular basis. Chapter 6 gives some delicious ways to fix sweet potatoes—and the recipes are also low in fat.

When researchers studied two groups of women in Singapore in 1977, they found that the group who ate a liberal amount of leafy green vegetables had a lower lung cancer rate than the women who did not include these foods in their diets. Dark green leafy vegetables made their intake of both vitamin C and beta-carotene (vitamin A) high.

- Cruciferous vegetables are also important on a cancer risk–reduction diet. They are part of the cabbage family—like broccoli, kale, turnips, brussels sprouts, and cauliflower. These vegetables contain natural substances called *indoles*. In laboratory studies, indoles have been shown to lower the risk for stomach and colon cancer.

Planning Vitamin-Rich Meals

Fruits and vegetables should be a main part of your daily diet—you need to move away from the typical "meat and potatoes" diet because it is too high in fat and too low in vitamins and fiber. Choose *at least* one vitamin-C-rich and one vitamin-A-rich fruit or vegetable, and one cruciferous vegetable every day. (See Appendix II for vitamin content of foods.) Make a list of your family's favorite vitamin-rich fruits and vegetables. Keep them well stocked in the refrigerator and serve generous portions with meals, especially if they are served without any added fat.

Here again, you can probably name many anticancer vegetables and fruits that are good for you, but you don't know what to do with them—foods like cabbage, kale, sweet potatoes, and turnips. With the recipes in this book, you can turn them into low-fat coleslaw, fritters, quiches, crudités, and desserts. To get the maximum benefit from these vitamin-rich dishes, check the introductions to Chapters 1 and 3, Appetizers and Salads. In them we suggest ways of handling and preparing vegetables and fruits so they don't lose their vitamin content.

I would like to emphasize again that the best way to ingest vitamins is through the whole foods that contain them, not through vitamin supplements. To date, no real evidence has linked low cancer incidence with vitamin supplements. In fact, vitamin A can be toxic in large, unmonitored doses of the synthetic form. But it is difficult to overdose on vitamin A–rich foods.

Eat more of the foods we just talked about. By eating more fruits, vegetables and whole grains, you will consume more fiber and vitamins. But also cut down on your intake of fat. If you have two vegetables, a piece of whole-grain bread, and fruit for dessert at a meal you will eat less meat (less fat), and still feel satisfied.

STEP 3: MINIMIZE INTAKE OF SALT-CURED OR SMOKED FOODS

The *Interim Guidelines* tell us to cut back on the amounts of salt-cured and smoked foods we eat.

Nitrates and Nitrites

The term *salt-cured* has nothing at all to do with the intake of table salt. Instead, it refers to a process of preserving foods like ham, bacon, sausage, and bologna that adds chemicals called *nitrates* or *nitrites* to prolong their shelf life and to keep the meat an attractive color. These chemicals combine with proteins (like those found in ham or bologna) to form powerful carcinogens (cancer-causing agents) called *nitrosamines*. These nitrosamines can form when cured meats like ham or bacon are simply eaten or when they are fried at high temperatures.

Studies done on Norwegians, who consume large quantities of salt-cured and smoked foods, have shown a high rate of stomach cancer. The researchers also found that when these Norwegians emigrated to the United States, and kept their same diet of smoked and salt-cured fish, their rate of cancer stayed high. Not only that, as some of their American neighbors started to eat this typical Norwegian food, the Americans' cancer rate also went up substantially.

Limit the use of ham, bacon, and sausages in your diet (they are also high in fat) and try substituting other foods in their place. We include a 21-day menu in Chapter 10 of this book. You

will find many good breakfast and lunch ideas there that don't
use fatty lunch meats or nitrite-high bacon.

However, if you can't live without ham, bacon, or bologna, at
least cut down on how often you eat it. First have it twice a week,
then once a week, then once every ten days, making sure you are
buying products with vitamin C added.

Studies have shown that vitamin C (ascorbic acid) *limits*
(although it doesn't entirely prevent) the conversion of nitrites
into nitrosamines. So if you do keep salt-cured foods like ham or
bacon in your diet, make sure you always include a vitamin-C-
rich fruit or vegetable with the meal, like tomatoes on a ham
sandwich or grapefruit with your bacon-and-pancakes
breakfast.

Some food manufacturers have begun adding vitamin C to
meat products that contain nitrites or nitrates. Even better,
others are producing ham, bacon, and sausages without these
offending chemicals. It is especially gratifying that baby foods
containing these meats—like "vegetable ham" or "vegetable
bacon dinner"—are *all* made *without* nitrates or nitrites. (Children don't consume these chemicals until they eat "adult" food!)

To find out which foods contain nitrates or nitrites, read the
label before you buy a product.

Smoked Foods—to Barbecue or Not to Barbecue?

Another question my patients constantly ask is: "What's wrong
with barbecueing—can it really cause cancer?"

When you barbecue, you are cooking food by smoking it.
Cancer-causing substances are formed when wood, paper, or
charcoal burns. These carcinogenic substances can be carried
up to your food by the smoke and flames. If you just love to
barbecue, you can help limit the presence of these carcinogens
by following a few suggestions:

- Broil in your oven with gas or electric heat, *under*—not
  over—the flames
- Brush food with Liquid Smoke—it gives the flavor of a
  barbecue without the carcinogens
- Remove the skin from chicken after it is charcoal-
  broiled—you are not only removing the fat but also
  taking off that part of the chicken that has been
  contaminated by smoke
- Cook meats as far away from flames or charcoal as
  possible

• Cover the coals with aluminum foil to prevent meat or other foods from being exposed to smoke or flames.

You can still enjoy cooking out or barbecueing. But keep it to an occasional treat and follow the cooking directions above.

STEP 4: DRINK ALCOHOL
ONLY IN MODERATION

This recommendation is pretty clear-cut. Moderation means no more than two alcoholic drinks per day—like a light wine with dinner. In addition to other health problems, heavy drinking—especially in conjunction with cigarette smoking—can lead to cancer of the mouth and cancer of the esophagus. And as the liver begins to deteriorate from excessive consumption of alcohol, it can sometimes become cancerous.

HOW TO USE THIS BOOK TO MAKE
YOUR DAILY FOOD CHOICES

You can see from the preceding four steps that in order to effectively adopt a cancer risk–reduction diet, you must moderate your intake of harmful substances like fat, nitrates, and alcohol, and increase your intake of vitamin- and fiber-rich whole foods like fruits, vegetables, and whole grains. The recipes in this book meet all these requirements. They will provide you with a delicious and varied diet that includes everything from appetizers to desserts, party menus, and holiday meals—culinary experiences that are both good-tasting and good for you.

How Much Food?

The first step in starting your cancer risk–reduction eating plan is to have a doctor or registered dietitian (nutritionist with an R.D.) figure your ideal weight and how many calories a day you should be consuming. This, of course, will vary with your level of activity. People who exercise vigorously can consume more calories than those who are less active. Then if you are in general good health, you can begin your eating plan right away. However, if you have a significant medical illness such as diabetes, first review this program with your physician or nutritionist.

Using the Recipes

Using an updated computer software program, we have analyzed each recipe in this book for the following per serving: calories, percent calories from fat, grams of fat, grams of fiber, amount of vitamin A (IU) and amount of vitamin C (milligrams). This way you can calculate exactly how much fat, fiber, and vitamins you are consuming when you use these recipes. In some of the recipes we give a choice of ingredients—for example, chicken breasts, or whole chicken cut into pieces. The recipe analysis is always based on the choice listed first (in this case, chicken breasts).

You will find important and interesting issues addressed in each of the chapter introductions, like

- how you can still enjoy cheese even though it is high-fat food
- how to make an elegant vitamin-rich soup in 10 minutes using leftover vegetables
- cooking times and procedures for making perfectly good vegetables without vitamin loss
- how to make a reduced-fat vinaigrette that doesn't taste watery or bland

For the sake of general good health, we have minimized the use of salt and cholesterol-laden foods, even though their ingestion is not specifically linked to cancer at this time.

How Effective Is This Plan?

I would like to emphasize that the recipes in this book are neither a cure for cancer nor a guarantee that you will not contract it. However, modifying your diet through the use of these recipes may help reduce your chances of developing cancer. I would also like to address the people who say that they will pay attention to what they eat only when there is positive proof that cancer can be prevented through diet. There was also a dubious group 20 years ago that said they would believe the connection between lung cancer and smoking when there was "positive proof." Sadly, many of them did not live to hear the proof that they wanted.

Positive thoughts are an overall good health rule. Think in terms of new foods/good foods, new experiences/good experiences—the good you are doing when you cook to prevent cancer.

We know you will find the recipes in this book delicious, innovative, and totally consistent with the National Research Council and the American Cancer Society recommendations. The recipes as well as the menus provided are only the beginning of the many possibilities of a solid cancer risk–reduction eating regimen. Once you know the principles of low-fat, high-fiber, and vitamin-rich cooking, eating to prevent cancer will become an enjoyable habit and you will form lifelong, healthful eating patterns.

Bon appétit!

1
Appetizers

Artichokes with Shrimp Salsa
Brussels Sprouts Frittata
Caponata
Chicken Puffs
Chicken Tumble in Lettuce Cups
Cottage Cheese Dip and Stuffing
Cucumber Dip
Fillet of Sole in Orange Marinade
Foil-Wrapped Chicken
Green Salsa
Hummus
Mini Vegetable Fritters
Mozzarella Vegetable Canapés
Oriental Meatballs
Party Mix

Red Salsa
Refried Bean Platter
Salmon Spread
Seafood Pâté
Spanish Bean Dip
Spiced Chicken Cubes
Spinach Dip
Stuffed Grape Leaves (Dolmas)
Tabbouleh Dip
Tortilla Chips
Tuna-Cheese Soufflés
Tuna Spread
*Turkey-Pineapple Brochettes with
    Peanut Sauce*
Vegetable Antipasto

Appetizers

If appetizers—in the traditional sense—are meant to entice and stimulate the palate for the rest of the meal, then we have adopted some bad habits with the kinds that we serve. Overrich and high-fat concoctions are too often the typical cocktail party fare.

A well-planned array of low-fat appetizers can taste scrumptious, beautify a table, and dazzle your guests with their diverse appeal. A perfect way to begin a party is to gather your friends around a beautifully executed vegetable platter. It incorporates many foods like carrots, cauliflower, broccoli, raw turnips, red and green peppers—that are high in either vitamin A, vitamin C, or both, and are also a good source of dietary fiber. These vegetables have a clean, crisp taste, require a minimum of preparation, and are relatively economical. Presented with delicious dips like Hummus, Cucumber Dip, Spinach Dip, or Caponata, their eye appeal and taste make them a sure favorite. You can even color-coordinate them for theme parties. Use red and green pepper strips interspersed with broccoli florets and cherry tomatoes on a pretty Christmas platter. Put creamy Cottage Cheese Dip in the center, sprinkle with a dash of paprika, and top with a sprig of parsley.

A few tips will ensure maximum enjoyment of these vegetable trays:

- If you have the time, check local produce stands and farmers' markets for seasonal vegetables. There is a difference in freshness, taste, and usually price, local products being cheaper.
- Do not destroy vitamins by poor storage and handling habits. When you bring your vegetables home, rinse them under cool water, pat dry, and store in an airtight plastic bag or container in the refrigerator. Some vitamin A can be lost by wilting or dehydration. Vitamin C is especially susceptible to excess heat and exposure to air, and is soluble in water.
- To make dense vegetables like broccoli, carrots, turnips, and cauliflower more chewable, you may wish to blanch them (drop into rapidly boiling water for about three minutes).
- As tempting as it might be in order to save time, don't precut your vegetables hours ahead of time. This can dry them out significantly and they will look shriveled. Make preparing the raw vegetable platter one of your last tasks before putting the party spread out for your guests.

There are many appetizers that can be made ahead of time without compromising taste or appearance. Stuffed Grape Leaves (Dolmas) is one—it is actually more flavorful if stored in the refrigerator overnight. This is a great finger food and can be served plain or with piquant Dill Sauce. Dolmas were one of civilization's first hors d'oeuvres. Served in the third century B.C. in Greece to visiting royalty, their longstanding popularity is a testimonial to their appeal. Tabbouleh Dip is another appetizer that stores well for a day or two; its flavor becomes richer with a little extra time.

For added elegance at your party, serve Salmon Spread with squares of rye or pumpernickel bread. And for an ethnic touch, pass around Oriental Meatballs or wedges of Brussels Sprouts Frittata.

You will notice in the recipe analysis that a few of the appetizers contain more than 30% calories from fat. Most traditional appetizers like cheese and pâtés are 75–85% calories from fat. While it is best to serve the appetizers with less than 30% calories from fat, in instances when the meal served is less than 30% calories from fat (or during special occasions) appetizers with higher fat content can be served.

In this chapter, we include a number of appetizers that contain cheese as one of the ingredients. Hard cheese has approximately 73% calories from fat and, for the most part, should be avoided in quantities more than a sprinkling. There are, however, a number of cheeses that are lower in fat and can be used moderately on a cancer risk–reduction diet. These include low-fat cottage cheese, part-skim ricotta, part-skim mozzarella, and part-skim feta cheese. (Always read labels to be sure. The first ingredient should say "part-skim or skim milk.") There are other cheeses that are lower in fat than regular cheeses, like low-fat cheddar or monterey jack, but they are usually higher in sodium and are harder to find in major supermarkets.

One popular reduced-fat cheese is neufchâtel cream cheese. We use this product in Salmon Spread. We halve the amount of cream cheese called for, use neufchâtel instead, and add unflavored gelatin to set the spread. The taste is still rich and creamy with 50% less fat.

Even using low-fat cheeses, we have kept the amounts to a minimum, using approximately 1 to 2 tablespoons grated cheese per person for a nonentrée dish and approximately ½ cup grated cheese per person for an entrée. We have included cheese in this book because it is a food some people just can't give up (the authors included). We have merely minimized the fat content without compromising taste.

It is important to remember that, for most people, milk products are a major source of calcium. This mineral is necessary for good health and is thought to be beneficial toward the prevention of osteoporosis. If you are substituting cheese for a milk serving, note that all it takes is 1 cup of yogurt, 2 cups low-fat cottage cheese, or 1⅓ ounces of natural cheese to equal 1 cup of milk. Use skim or low-fat milk products whenever possible; the amount of calcium per serving remains basically the same.

In several of the following recipes, food items are marinated in oil-containing mixtures for several hours or overnight. Don't be alarmed by the large amounts of oil used; less than a third to a half of the mixture will actually be eaten. But it is still important to use marinades that are lower in fat, because when regular oil-containing mixtures are used to marinate and baste meats, about ½ teaspoon of fat is added per ounce of meat. With a 3- to 4-ounce portion, the fat adds up fast.

Appetizers can also be a leisurely first course at a more formal dinner party. Again, you don't want to stuff your guests—you want them to look forward to the rest of the meal. Two elegant and light first courses in this chapter are Fillet of Sole in Orange

Marinade and Seafood Pâté. Both are examples of excellent flavor, texture, and spice combinations. They demonstrate how easy it is to excite the palate without filling up the stomach.

Finally, we suggest that you be as fanciful and creative as you wish. Please yourself as well as your guests; your reputation as a host or hostess can only be enhanced.

ARTICHOKES WITH SHRIMP SALSA

4 ounces small cooked shrimp

1 large tomato, peeled, seeded, and chopped (to peel and seed, see page 224)

½ green bell pepper, chopped

2 scallions, sliced

1½ tablespoons fresh cilantro (coriander)

1 tablespoon diced mild green chilies (canned)

1½ teaspoons lemon juice

1 clove garlic, minced

¼ teaspoon oregano

⅛ teaspoon ground cumin

⅛ teaspoon pepper

1 large or 2 medium artichokes, cooked

Combine all ingredients except artichokes. Let set in refrigerator for at least 2 hours to allow flavors to develop.

Carefully remove leaves from artichoke and pick out the 36 best ones. Place approximately 1 tablespoon of the salsa on each artichoke leaf. Arrange on a platter and serve.

Makes 36 hors d'oeuvres

NUTRITIVE VALUES PER HORS D'OEUVRE

FAT	FIBER	VIT. A	VIT. C	CAL	CAL FROM FAT
.27gm	1.48gm	344 IU	17.8mg	28	9%

BRUSSELS SPROUTS FRITTATA

A great appetizer—at home or on a picnic.

1 10-ounce package frozen brussels sprouts
⅓ cup finely chopped onion
⅓ cup finely chopped green bell pepper
2 cloves garlic, minced
2 tablespoons chicken broth
¼ cup wheat germ
½ teaspoon salt
¼ teaspoon pepper
½ teaspoon oregano
3 drops tabasco sauce (hot pepper sauce)
⅓ cup chopped parsley
¼ pound part-skim mozzarella cheese, grated
1 egg, lightly beaten
2 egg whites
2 tablespoons parmesan cheese, grated
2 tablespoons bread crumbs (dried)
Paprika

Steam sprouts until they are just done. Drain and coarsely chop. Sauté onion, bell pepper, and garlic in broth for 5 minutes. Remove from heat. Add chopped brussels sprouts, wheat germ, salt, pepper, oregano, tabasco, parsley, and mozzarella cheese. Stir in the whole egg.

Stiffly beat egg whites and gently fold into remaining mixture, only until blended—don't overmix. Transfer to an 8-inch-square pan lightly coated with cooking spray, and gently smooth top. Mix parmesan and bread crumbs and sprinkle over the frittata. Sprinkle with paprika and bake in a preheated oven at 325°F for 30 minutes. Cool a bit and cut into 36 squares. May be served hot or at room temperature.

Makes 36 squares

NUTRITIVE VALUES PER SQUARE:

FAT	FIBER	VIT. A	VIT. C	CAL	CAL FROM FAT
.85mg	.38mg	134 IU	10.5mg	19.6	39%

CAPONATA

Serve this zesty eggplant appetizer with whole-wheat toast squares and raw vegetables for dipping. Any leftover Caponata freezes well.

2 tablespoons olive oil
2 cups finely chopped celery
¾ cup finely chopped onions
2 tablespoons corn or safflower oil
2 pounds eggplant, peeled and cut in very small cubes
⅓ cup red wine vinegar
1 tablespoon sugar
3 cups finely chopped fresh tomatoes (or canned
    tomatoes, drained, if fresh unavailable)
2 tablespoons tomato paste
6 black olives, chopped
2 tablespoons capers
1 ounce flat anchovies, rinsed and chopped
¼ teaspoon pepper

WHOLE-WHEAT TOAST SQUARES
24 slices whole-wheat bread, quartered

Heat olive oil. Add celery and onions and sauté over moderate heat for 10 minutes. Transfer to a bowl. Add corn or safflower oil to the same saucepan and sauté eggplant over medium-high heat for 6–8 minutes, until softened. Return onions and celery to pan and add vinegar, sugar, tomatoes, tomato paste, black olives, capers, anchovies, and pepper. Simmer, uncovered, for 20 minutes. If desired, add more pepper or vinegar, or a bit of salt.

Run through a food processor or blender slightly—just to break up large pieces. Don't puree, as some texture is desirable. Serve at room temperature. Dry bread quarters in a 250°F oven for 30 minutes. Cool and serve with Caponata.

Makes 8 cups/Serves 24

NUTRITIVE VALUES PER SERVING (¼ cup):

FAT	FIBER	VIT. A	VIT. C	CAL	CAL FROM FAT
3.81gm	3.97gm	386 IU	9.48mg	129	27%

CHICKEN PUFFS

These are elegant, but easy to prepare.

½ cup cooked, finely minced chicken
1½ tablespoons mayonnaise
1 tablespoon dry bread crumbs
¼ teaspoon salt
¼ teaspoon dry mustard
½ teaspoon curry powder
¼ teaspoon worcestershire sauce
2 teaspoons minced scallions
1 egg white
24 whole-wheat toast squares, using 6 slices
    bread
Paprika

Mix all ingredients except egg white, toast squares, and paprika. This can be done several hours ahead and refrigerated.

To prepare toast squares, quarter bread slices and dry in a 250°F oven for 30 minutes. Just before serving Chicken Puffs, stiffly beat egg white and gently fold it into the chicken mixture. Mound on toast squares or crackers. Sprinkle with paprika and bake in a preheated 500°F oven for 5 minutes. Serve immediately.

Makes 24 puffs

NUTRITIVE VALUES PER PUFF:

FAT	FIBER	VIT. A	VIT. C	CAL	CAL FROM FAT
1.08gm	.443gm	6.76 IU	.055mg	33.7	29%

CHICKEN TUMBLE
IN LETTUCE CUPS

12 medium leaves of butter lettuce
1 tablespoon corn or safflower oil
½ pound minced raw chicken breast
2 chopped scallions
¼ cup sliced water chestnuts
2 tablespoons soy sauce
¼ cup chicken broth
1 tablespoon cornstarch
2 tablespoons water

Gently wash lettuce leaves and carefully dry them well with a towel, keeping them whole. You may need 2 heads of lettuce to get 12 leaves that are not torn. Heat oil in a frying pan and add chicken. Sauté until browned, separating pieces of chicken while sautéing. Add scallions, water chestnuts, soy sauce, and broth. Simmer for 5 minutes. Mix cornstarch with water, add to chicken mixture, and cook over medium-high heat until sauce thickens a bit.

Immediately transfer chicken mixture to a serving bowl set on a large tray or platter. Place the lettuce leaves on the platter surrounding the bowl. Each person takes a lettuce leaf, spoons in some chicken mixture, and folds the leaf to form a square packet. Napkins will be greatly appreciated!

Serves 12 as an hors d'oeuvre or 4 as an entrée

NUTRITIVE VALUES PER SERVING:

FAT	FIBER	VIT. A	VIT. C	CAL	CAL FROM FAT
1.72gm	.42gm	135 IU	1.96mg	42	37%

COTTAGE CHEESE
DIP AND STUFFING

1 cup low-fat cottage cheese
1 tablespoon fresh lemon juice
¼ teaspoon dried dill weed
1 scallion, finely chopped
¼ teaspoon pepper
¼ teaspoon salt
2 tablespoons buttermilk
1 tablespoon mayonnaise
24 whole-wheat crackers
3 carrots, cut into 8 sticks each
Cherry tomatoes (optional)

Mix all ingredients (except crackers and vegetables) in blender or food processor until very smooth. Serve as a dip with crackers and carrot sticks, or to stuff cherry tomatoes.

Makes 1½ cups/Serves 6

NUTRITIVE VALUES PER SERVING:

FAT	FIBER	VIT. A	VIT. C	CAL	CAL FROM FAT
4.86gm	3.10gm	4108 IU	4.91mg	130	34%

CUCUMBER DIP

This could also be served as a refreshing accompaniment for spicy dishes such as curry.

> 1 teaspoon salt
> 2 large cucumbers, peeled and grated
> 2 cloves garlic, minced
> 1 cup low-fat yogurt
> 1 tablespoon mayonnaise
> 2 scallions, chopped
> ½ cup chopped watercress
> ¼ teaspoon pepper
> ¼ teaspoon celery seed
> 3 cups broccoli florets
> 3 whole carrots, each cut into 8 sticks

Sprinkle salt over grated cucumbers and let stand for 30 minutes. Squeeze out moisture with hands. Let stand another 15 minutes, and squeeze again to get cucumbers as moisture-free as possible.

Mix cucumbers with all remaining ingredients except broccoli and carrots. Dip broccoli and carrots into the Cucumber Dip.

Makes 3 cups/Serves 10

NUTRITIVE VALUES PER SERVING:

FAT	FIBER	VIT. A	VIT. C	CAL	CAL FROM FAT
1.88gm	3.16gm	3178 IU	35mg	44.3	38%

FILLET OF SOLE
IN ORANGE MARINADE

An elegant first course.

1 pound sole fillets (or other boneless white fish fillets)

1 cup fish stock, or ½ cup chicken stock plus ½ cup water

¼ cup corn or safflower oil

2 tablespoons white wine vinegar

¼ cup orange juice

½ teaspoon salt

⅛ teaspoon cayenne pepper

¼ cup slivered green bell pepper

¼ cup finely sliced scallions

1 carrot, grated

1 orange, peeled and cut into 6 slices

Gently simmer fish in stock over medium heat for 3 minutes on each side or until barely done. Discard stock or save for other uses.

Make a marinade of all remaining ingredients except orange slices. Arrange fish in a serving dish (or on individual plates) and pour marinade over fish, being sure to include some vegetables on each portion.

Marinate in refrigerator for several hours. Before serving, pour excess marinade off fish, and garnish each serving with an orange slice. Serve chilled.

Serves 6

NUTRITIVE VALUES PER SERVING:

FAT	FIBER	VIT. A	VIT. C	CAL	CAL FROM FAT
5.29gm	1.28gm	1499 IU	23.5mg	113	42%

FOIL-WRAPPED CHICKEN

1 tablespoon corn or safflower oil

2 tablespoons soy sauce

3 tablespoons finely chopped fresh cilantro (coriander)

4 cloves garlic, minced

4 scallions, finely chopped

¼ cup hoisin sauce (found in Oriental section of market)

1 pound boneless chicken breast, cut in 60 pieces

Make marinade by combining all ingredients except chicken. Add chicken pieces to marinade and marinate for several hours, stirring a few times.

Stir chicken and marinade to distribute sauce and vegetables among chicken pieces.

Place each piece of marinade-coated chicken on a 4-inch square of foil, including whatever sauce and vegetables adhere to each piece. Fold foil in half over chicken, so that edges are even. Fold each of the open 3 edges 2 or 3 times to make an airtight package. Place chicken packets on a baking sheet. Bake in a preheated 350°F oven for 15 minutes. Serve in packets.

Makes 60 packets

NUTRITIVE VALUES PER PACKET:

FAT	FIBER	VIT. A	VIT. C	CAL	CAL FROM FAT
.43gm	.02gm	17.8 IU	.27mg	11.6	33%

GREEN SALSA

A delicious and colorful variation of the better-known red salsa, it is excellent as a dip for tortilla chips, or as a sauce for enchiladas, tacos, or any other Mexican dish.

1 13-ounce can Mexican green tomatoes
    (tomatillos), drained and chopped
⅓ cup finely chopped onions
¼ cup chopped fresh cilantro (coriander)
1 tablespoon corn or safflower oil
1½ teaspoons diced mild green chilies (canned)
1 clove garlic, minced
¼ teaspoon salt
⅛ teaspoon pepper
⅛ teaspoon sugar
6 flour tortillas, made into chips (see Tortilla
    Chips)

Blend all ingredients except tortillas in food processor or blender. Don't puree, as some texture is desirable.

May be served chilled or at room temperature.

Makes 2 cups/Serves 6

Nutritive Values per Serving:

FAT	FIBER	VIT. A	VIT. C	CAL	CAL FROM FAT
4.2gm	1.26gm	563 IU	11.8mg	131	29%

HUMMUS

A Middle Eastern garbanzo bean dip with a wonderful hint of lemon.

- ¼ cup sesame seeds, toasted
- 1 15-ounce can garbanzo beans, drained (save liquid)
- ½ teaspoon salt
- ⅛ teaspoon pepper
- 3 cloves garlic, minced
- ¼ cup fresh lemon juice
- 3 tablespoons olive oil
- 1 tablespoon liquid from drained beans
- 4 slices pita bread, each cut or torn into 6–8 triangles
- 3 carrots, each cut into 8 sticks

Heat sesame seeds over medium heat in an ungreased frying pan for 5 minutes or until light golden brown, tossing seeds several times while toasting. Blend toasted sesame seeds, garbanzo beans, salt, pepper, garlic, lemon juice, oil, and 1 tablespoon liquid in food processor or blender to make a smooth puree. Add more bean liquid if mixture is too thick to scoop up with pita bread. Serve as a dip for the pita bread and carrot sticks.

Makes 3 cups/Serves 8

Nutritive Values per Serving:

FAT	FIBER	VIT. A	VIT. C	CAL	CAL FROM FAT
9.39gm	5.63gm	3036 IU	5.79mg	260	33%

MINI VEGETABLE FRITTERS

Somewhat like potato-pancakes—but these small fritters have much more flavor.

2 eggs, beaten
1½ cups grated unpeeled potatoes
1 cup grated carrots
¼ cup finely chopped onion
¼ cup finely chopped green bell pepper
3 tablespoons unbleached white flour
½ teaspoon oregano
⅛ teaspoon cayene pepper
¼ teaspoon worcestershire sauce
½ teaspoon salt
1 tablespoon corn or safflower oil

Combine all ingredients except oil and mix well. Brush nonstick pan lightly with a bit of the oil. For each fritter, spoon 1 tablespoon vegetable mixture onto a medium-hot pan. Flatten fritters and cook for about 3 minutes, or until golden brown on each side.

Brush pan with more oil as needed to cook remaining fritters. Keep cooked fritters warm on baking sheet, in a single layer, until all are cooked. May be recrisped by heating in the center of a 400°F oven for 5 minutes.

Makes 36 fritters

NUTRITIVE VALUES PER SERVING:

FAT	FIBER	VIT. A	VIT. C	CAL	CAL FROM FAT
.71gm	.382gm	355 IU	3.42mg	19.7	33%

MOZZARELLA-VEGETABLE CANAPES

½ cup finely chopped carrots
½ cup finely chopped radishes
¼ cup finely chopped onions
2 tablespoons finely chopped green bell pepper
1 garlic clove, minced
2 tablespoons mayonnaise
1 tablespoon low-fat yogurt
½ teaspoon salt
¼ teaspoon pepper
48 small Rye Crisp crackers or melba rounds
4 ounces part-skim mozzarella cheese, cut in 48
    small slices
Paprika

Mix all ingredients except crackers, cheese, and paprika. Spread approximately ½ tablespoon of mixture on each cracker and cover with a small slice of mozzarella cheese. Sprinkle with paprika. Bake at 500°F for 5 minutes and serve immediately.

Makes 48 canapés

Nutritive Values per Canape:

FAT	FIBER	VIT. A	VIT. C	CAL	CAL FROM FAT
.948gm	.832gm	144 IU	1.06mg	33.2	26%

ORIENTAL MEATBALLS

1 pound ground round

2 10-ounce packages frozen chopped spinach, defrosted and squeezed dry (save liquid for other uses)

2 tablespoons soy sauce

1 tablespoon sherry

1 tablespoon sesame oil (found in Oriental section of market)

$1\frac{1}{2}$ tablespoons cornstarch

2 scallions, finely chopped (about $\frac{1}{3}$ cup)

1 egg, slightly beaten

1 cup dry bread crumbs

2 teaspoons corn or safflower oil

Mix all ingredients except 2 teaspoons corn oil, and form into 36 meatballs. Spread corn oil on a baking sheet. Place meatballs on sheet and bake at 350°F for 10 minutes. Shake pan to turn meatballs, and drain off liquid. Bake 5 minutes more. Lift out of pan with a slotted spoon, draining off liquid.

May be served alone, or with Ginger Sauce or Sweet and Sour Sauce (see index).

Makes 36 meatballs

NUTRITIVE VALUES PER MEATBALL

FAT	FIBER	VIT. A	VIT. C	CAL	CAL FROM FAT
1.95gm	.94gm	1268 IU	3.21mg	43.4	41%

PARTY MIX

1 cube margarine or butter

2 tablespoons soy sauce

2 tablespoons worcestershire sauce

$\frac{1}{2}$ teaspoon garlic powder

2 cups Rice Chex

2 cups Corn Chex

2 cups Bran Chex

2 cups Wheat Chex

1 11-ounce bag unsalted pretzel sticks

Melt margarine in a large baking pan in a preheated 300°F oven. Add the soy sauce, worcestershire sauce, and garlic powder. Gently toss the cereals with the margarine mixture, two cups at a time until evenly coated. When thoroughly mixed, add pretzel sticks and bake at 300°F for 1 hour, stirring every 15 minutes. Cool before serving. If you don't have a large baking pan with fairly high sides, you will probably find it easier to use 2 baking pans.

Makes 12 cups/36 servings

NUTRITIVE VALUES PER SERVING:

FAT	FIBER	VIT. A	VIT. C	CAL	CAL FROM FAT
3.02gm	.89gm	119 IU	4.35mg	87.0	31%

RED SALSA

As well as being a wonderful sauce in which to dip tortilla chips, it is an excellent way to add interest to plain broiled chicken or meat or to vegetarian dishes.

1½ cups fresh tomatoes, coarsely chopped (or drained canned tomatoes, if fresh are unavailable)

¼ cup finely chopped scallions

2 tablespoons chopped fresh cilantro (coriander)

1 tablespoon corn or safflower oil

2 tablespoons diced mild green chilies (canned)

1 clove garlic, minced

¼ teaspoon salt

⅛ teaspoon pepper

⅛ teaspoon sugar

1 tablespoon red wine vinegar

6 flour tortillas, made into chips (see Tortilla Chips)

Put all ingredients except tortillas through blender or food processor until coarsely chopped. Don't puree, as some texture is desirable. May be served chilled or at room temperature.

Makes 2 cups/Serves 6

NUTRITIVE VALUES PER SERVING:

FAT	FIBER	VIT. A	VIT. C	CAL	CAL FROM FAT
4.2gm	2.18gm	705 IU	17.7mg	134	28%

REFRIED BEAN PLATTER

1 17-ounce can refried beans (vegetarian, if available)

4 ounces part-skim mozzarella cheese, grated

2 tablespoons low-fat yogurt

2 tablespoons sour cream

1 medium-sized avocado, chopped

½ cup chopped radishes (about 10)

4 scallions, sliced (about ½ cup)

2 medium tomatoes, chopped (about 1 cup)

3 flour tortillas, made into chips (see Tortilla Chips)

2½ carrots, cut into 20 sticks

Preheat oven to 350°F.

Spread refried beans evenly on a 10-inch ovenproof plate. Top with grated cheese, and heat in a 350°F oven for 15 minutes.

Combine yogurt and sour cream. Remove beans from oven and add toppings in this order:

yogurt-sour cream mixture in the center,

circle of chopped avocado around the sour cream,

circle of radishes around the chopped avocado,

circle of scallions around the radishes, and

circle of tomatoes around the scallions.

Serve with Tortilla Chips and carrot sticks, scooping from the outside to the center to get a taste of all toppings.

Serves 8–10

NUTRITIVE VALUES PER SERVING:

FAT	FIBER	VIT. A	VIT. C	CAL	CAL FROM FAT
8.52gm	7.16gm	3783 IU	13.6mg	185	41%

SALMON SPREAD

1 envelope unflavored gelatin (1 tablespoon)

½ cup boiling water

4 ounces low-fat cream cheese (neufchâtel), cut
   in several pieces

2 tablespoons mayonnaise

1 tablespoon white wine vinegar

1 8-ounce can salmon, drained and flaked with
   a fork

½ cup finely chopped green bell pepper

12 pimiento-stuffed green olives, chopped

Paprika

1 small bunch parsley, separated into sprigs

2 tablespoons capers

10 cherry tomatoes, halved

10 slices pumpernickel bread, quartered

Dissolve gelatin in ½ cup boiling water. Put in food processor or
blender with cream cheese and mix until very smooth. Add
mayonnaise, vinegar, salmon, green bell pepper, and olives. Mix
just until blended; some texture is desirable. Pour into a 3-cup
mold or bowl. Refrigerate several hours until set.

Unmold and sprinkle with paprika. Decorate with parsley,
capers, and cherry tomatoes. Serve quartered slices of pumpernickel bread with the spread.

Serves 10

NUTRITIVE VALUES PER SERVING:

FAT	FIBER	VIT. A	VIT. C	CAL	CAL FROM FAT
7.16gm	2.7gm	353 IU	14.1mg	169	38%

SEAFOOD PATE

1½ pounds fillet of sole
2 egg whites
1 cup low-fat milk
½ teaspoon salt
½ teaspoon paprika
¼ teaspoon white pepper
½ teaspoon tarragon
¼ cup minced onion
1 cup watercress, chopped
1 additional bunch watercress for garnish
16 cherry tomatoes for garnish

MUSTARD SAUCE

3 tablespoons mayonnaise
3 tablespoons low-fat yogurt
3 tablespoons low-fat milk
1½ teaspoons dijon mustard
1½ teaspoons capers, drained
1 teaspoon tarragon

In processor or blender, puree fish until smooth. Add egg whites, one at a time, blending well after each addition. Add milk, ⅓ cup at a time, processing mixture just enough to blend after each addition. Transfer fish mixture to a bowl and gently fold in salt, paprika, pepper, tarragon, onion and chopped watercress, keeping mixture light in texture.

Gently spoon fish mixture into a loaf pan coated with cooking spray, gently smooth the top, and cover with foil. Place in a larger baking pan; add enough hot water to come halfway up the sides. Bake for 1 hour in a preheated 375°F oven.

Cool for 5 minutes before unmolding. Tip pan to drain liquid (there will be a lot). Invert onto a serving platter. Garnish with additional watercress and tomatoes. Pâté may also be sliced into 8 servings, dished onto individual plates, and garnished.

To prepare mustard sauce, stir all sauce ingredients together until smooth. Spoon some sauce over the fish and pass the rest.

Serves 8 as a first course

NUTRITIVE VALUES PER SERVING:

FAT	FIBER	VIT. A	VIT. C	CAL	CAL FROM FAT
5.61gm	.65gm	464 IU	9.48mg	124	41%

SPANISH BEAN DIP

Serve with baked Tortilla Chips (see Index) and raw vegetables for scooping—try carrots, jicama, radishes, green onions, and cherry tomatoes for a delectable variety of color and texture.

1 17-ounce can refried beans (vegetarian, if available)
4 ounces part-skim mozzarella cheese, grated
4 scallions, sliced
¼ cup diced mild green chilies (canned)
1 teaspoon chili powder
¼ cup sour cream
¼ cup low-fat yogurt

Mix all ingredients together in a saucepan until well blended. Heat gently over medium heat for 10 minutes, stirring often. Serve hot or at room temperature.

Makes 3 cups/Serves 12

NUTRITIVE VALUES PER SERVING:

FAT	FIBER	VIT. A	VIT. C	CAL	CAL FROM FAT
3.84gm	3.92gm	1096 IU	7.3mg	88.4	39%

SPICED CHICKEN CUBES

½ medium onion, chopped

3 cloves garlic, minced

2 tablespoons corn or safflower oil

2 tablespoons red wine vinegar

2 tablespoons catsup

1½ teaspoons ground cumin

1½ teaspoons paprika

¼ teaspoon pepper

1 teaspoon ground coriander

¼ teaspoon powdered ginger

⅛ teaspoon cayenne pepper

1½ pounds boneless chicken or turkey breast,
   raw, cut into 48 pieces

2 8-ounce cans whole water chestnuts, drained
   and cut in half

48 toothpicks

Lettuce leaves

Mix onion, garlic, oil, vinegar, catsup, cumin, paprika, pepper, coriander, ginger, and cayenne pepper together to make a marinade. Add chicken pieces to the marinade and marinate for several hours. Place each chicken piece on a toothpick with a water chestnut half. Bake in marinade for 10 minutes at 350°F. Drain off marinade and serve chicken on a platter lined with lettuce leaves.

Makes 48 cubes

NUTRITIVE VALUES PER CUBE:

FAT	FIBER	VIT. A	VIT. C	CAL	CAL FROM FAT
.68gm	.33gm	7.57 IU	.24mg	23.1	26%

SPINACH DIP

2 10-ounce packages frozen chopped spinach,
   defrosted and squeezed dry
¼ cup mayonnaise
½ cup buttermilk
½-¾ teaspoon pepper*
⅓ cup finely sliced scallions
1 garlic clove, minced
48 whole-grain crackers
48 carrot sticks (6 carrots, each cut into 8
   sticks)

Drain spinach and squeeze out liquid until it is very dry (if
spinach is not dry enough, the dip will be runny). Save liquid for
soup.

Using a fork, mix spinach with mayonnaise until fluffy, then
add buttermilk, pepper, scallions, and garlic and mix until well
blended. Serve with whole-grain crackers and raw carrot sticks.

*If you like a peppery flavor, you might want to use ¾ teaspoon
pepper, but start with ½ teaspoon and then taste before adding
more.

Makes 3 cups/Serves 8

NUTRITIVE VALUES PER SERVING:

FAT	FIBER	VIT. A	VIT. C	CAL	CAL FROM FAT
9.21gm	8.75gm	11,758 IU	19.5mg	189	44%

STUFFED GRAPE LEAVES (DOLMAS)

2 tablespoons olive oil
1 cup minced onion
1 carrot, grated
2 cloves garlic, minced
¼ cup sliced almonds
2 cups cooked brown rice (about ⅔ cup raw)
2 tablespoons fresh mint, or 1 teaspoon dried
    mint
Juice of ½ lemon
¼ cup chopped parsley
¼ teaspoon salt
⅛ teaspoon pepper
1 8-ounce jar grape leaves

COOKING LIQUID

2 cups water
¼ cup fresh lemon juice
¼ cup chicken or vegetable broth

Heat olive oil over medium-high heat. Sauté onion, carrot, and garlic in oil for 5 minutes. Add almonds, rice, mint, lemon juice, parsley, salt, and pepper and gently mix. Remove from heat.

Remove grape leaves from jar and separate carefully. Place a spoonful of the rice mixture at the base of each leaf. Roll up into tight bundles, tucking in sides, so they don't come apart while baking. Place, seam side down, in a baking pan where they fit as snugly as possible. Combine water, lemon juice, and broth to make the cooking liquid. Pour enough cooking liquid to cover grape leaves ¾ of the way up. Cover pan with foil and bake at 350°F for 1 hour and 15 minutes. Cool and serve.

Makes 48–60 dolmas

NUTRITIVE VALUES PER DOLMA:

FAT	FIBER	VIT. A	VIT. C	CAL	CAL FROM FAT
1.84gm	.37gm	105 IU	2.07mg	18.1	42%

TABBOULEH DIP

This makes an unusual appetizer, and can also be served as a salad or side dish for 6–8 people.

1 cup cracked wheat (bulgur)

2 cups cold water

2 medium ripe tomatoes

4 scallions, finely chopped

1½ cups chopped parsley

2 tablespoons fresh mint, or 1 teaspoon dried mint

3 tablespoons olive oil

5 tablespoons fresh lemon juice

¼ cup vegetable or chicken broth

½ teaspoon salt

¼ teaspoon pepper

20 small romaine lettuce leaves, washed, dried, and refrigerated to crisp

Soak bulgur in 2 cups cold water for 30 minutes. Drain very well so the dip will not be watery. Cut tomatoes in half, horizontally; squeeze out seeds and chop tomatoes.

Mix bulgur and tomatoes with all remaining ingredients except lettuce leaves. Refrigerate for several hours to allow flavors to develop.

Place bulgur mixture in a serving bowl placed on a platter. Surround serving bowl with the lettuce leaves, which are used to scoop up a portion of the Tabbouleh Dip.

Serves 10

NUTRITIVE VALUES PER SERVING:

FAT	FIBER	VIT. A	VIT. C	CAL	CAL FROM FAT
4.52gm	3.3gm	1456 IU	29.6mg	112	36%

TORTILLA CHIPS

These chips are just as good as the commercial ones, but without the unnecessary extra oil and salt.

3 flour tortillas

Liberally coat a baking sheet with cooking spray. Place the tortillas on the sheet; press down on them to get a light coating of the cooking spray on each one. Turn tortillas over and press down on other side.

Remove tortillas from baking sheet and cut each one into 10 triangles. Place triangles back on baking sheet in a single layer, and bake for 15 minutes in a preheated 350°F oven.

Makes 30 chips (3 servings of 10 each)

Nutritive Values per Serving:

FAT	FIBER	VIT. A	VIT. C	CAL	CAL FROM FAT
1.80gm	.57gm	2 IU	0mg	95	17%

TUNA-CHEESE SOUFFLES

1 7-ounce can white or albacore tuna in water (drained)
¼ cup parsley, chopped
¼ cup onion, chopped
2 tablespoons mayonnaise
6 green olives, chopped
1 tablespoon fresh lemon juice
¼ teaspoon pepper
3 egg whites
36 whole-wheat toast squares, using 9 slices bread
3 tablespoons freshly grated parmesan cheese
3 tablespoons dry bread crumbs
Paprika

Mix tuna, parsley, onion, mayonnaise, olives, lemon juice, and pepper in blender or food processor until smooth. Beat egg whites until stiff; gently fold into tuna mixture.

To make toast squares, quarter bread slices and dry in a 250°F oven for 30 minutes. Mound tuna mixture on toast squares. Combine parmesan cheese and bread crumbs and sprinkle on soufflés, then sprinkle with paprika. Heat under a preheated broiler for 5 minutes, or until lightly browned and slightly puffy. Serve at once.

Makes 36 soufflés

NUTRITIVE VALUES PER SOUFFLE:

FAT	FIBER	VIT. A	VIT. C	CAL	CAL FROM FAT
1.31gm	.516gm	30.6 IU	.769mg	41.3	29%

TUNA SPREAD

2 7-ounce cans white or albacore tuna in water
4 ounces low-fat cream cheese (neufchâtel), cut into 6 pieces
2 tablespoons mayonnaise
2 tablespoons fresh lemon juice
¼ cup sliced scallions
¼ teaspoon cayenne pepper
½ cup chopped parsley
1 tablespoon soy sauce
1 tablespoon sherry
12 whole-grain crackers
24 celery sticks
24 cucumber slices

Drain tuna. In blender or food processor, mix tuna until broken up. Add cream cheese, mayonnaise, lemon juice, scallions, cayenne pepper, parsley, soy sauce, and sherry, and mix until fairly smooth; don't puree, as some texture is desirable.

Refrigerate until slightly thickened, about 1 hour. Place in bowl in center of a large plate or platter and surround with whole-grain crackers and vegetable slices.

Serves 12

NUTRITIVE VALUES PER SERVING:

FAT	FIBER	VIT. A	VIT. C	CAL	CAL FROM FAT
4.83gm	1.81gm	426 IU	8.61mg	104	42%

TURKEY-PINEAPPLE BROCHETTES WITH PEANUT SAUCE

These freeze well, and may also be used as one dish in a Chinese meal or as a light entrée (serve with rice and salad).

SAUCE

1 tablespoon ground coriander
1 teaspoon salt
¼ teaspoon pepper
1 cup onion, chopped
2 cloves garlic, minced
⅓ cup soy sauce
¼ cup fresh lime juice (lemon juice may be substituted)
½ cup peanut butter
¼ cup brown sugar
⅓ cup oil

BROCHETTES

3 pounds boneless turkey or chicken breast, cut into 100 pieces
3 20-ounce cans pineapple chunks in juice, drained
100 toothpicks
1 bunch parsley

Combine sauce ingredients in a processor or blender. Marinate turkey pieces in sauce for several hours.

Put one marinated turkey cube and one pineapple chunk on each toothpick. Place brochettes on a baking pan with sides, cover with sauce, and bake at 350°F for 10 minutes. When done, lift turkey cubes out of sauce with slotted spoon. Serve on a platter lined with parsley.

Makes 100 brochettes

NUTRITIVE VALUES PER BROCHETTE:

FAT	FIBER	VIT. A	VIT. C	CAL	CAL FROM FAT
1.06gm	.39gm	54.4 IU	2.50mg	33.7	28%

VEGETABLE ANTIPASTO

MARINADE

½ cup olive oil
½ cup water
Juice of 2 lemons
2 bay leaves
2 garlic cloves, minced
8 whole peppercorns
½ teaspoon salt
1 tablespoon sugar

VEGETABLES

½ pound carrots, washed and cut into ¾-inch
   pieces
1 basket of cherry tomatoes, washed
1 10-ounce basket brussels sprouts, washed, or
   1 10-ounce package, frozen
Mustard greens or lettuce leaves

Mix marinade ingredients and bring to a boil. Simmer 15 minutes. Strain; divide into thirds. Simmer carrots in ⅓ of marinade for 10 minutes. Cool in marinade, then refrigerate in marinade. Simmer cherry tomatoes in second third of marinade for 5 minutes. Cool in marinade, then refrigerate in marinade.

Trim fresh brussels sprouts, and make an *X* in each root. Add 1 tablespoon sugar to last third of marinade and simmer brussels sprouts, fresh or still frozen, for 10 minutes, or until tender when pierced with a knife. Cool in marinade, then refrigerate in marinade.

To serve, lift each vegetable out of marinade and arrange attractively on platter lined with greenery. Accompany with toothpicks.

Serves 10

NUTRITIVE VALUES PER SERVING:

FAT	FIBER	VIT. A	VIT. C	CAL	CAL FROM FAT
2.82gm	3.13gm	3081 IU	40.1mg	52.9	48%

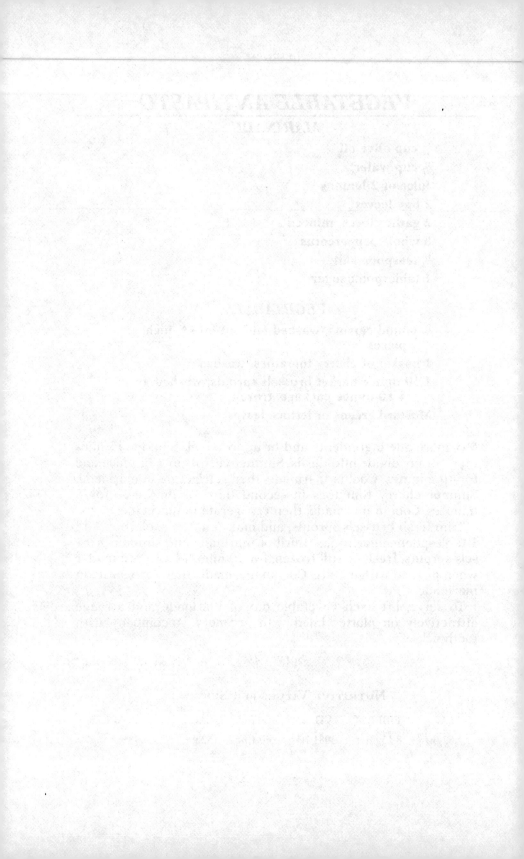

2
Soups

Beef Broth
Cabbage Soup
Chicken Chowder
Chicken Gumbo
Chilled Fresh Tomato Soup
Chinese Chicken Noodle Soup
Chinese Watercress and Cabbage Soup
Corn Chowder with Tomatoes
Cream of Broccoli Soup
Cream of Brussels Sprouts Soup
Creamy Vegetable Soup
Curried Carrot Soup
Egg-Lemon Soup
Fish Stock
French Onion Soup
Fresh Fish Soup

Gazpacho
Hot and Sour Soup
Lamb and Vegetable Soup
Lentil Soup
New England Seafood Chowder
Potato and Leek Soup with Carrots
Pumpkin Soup in a Shell
Spinach Soup
Tomato Bouillon
Tomato Soup
Vegetable Basil Soup
Vegetable Broth
Vegetable Soup with Pasta
Vichyssoise
White Bean and Spinach Soup
White Stock

Soups

Clear, creamy, or crunchy; sweet or spicy; thick or thin; hot or cold—soup can be fashioned to please every appetite. This wonderful food has been praised for its soothing effects both physical and psychological—chicken soup for the sniffles, tomato soup for the blues. The word *soup* itself conjures up images of steamy nourishment, good sustenance, and pleasant dining. Every nationality boasts its favorites, from miso, minestrone, and gazpacho to bouillabaisse, Scotch broth, and borscht.

Soup can be the perfect food on a cancer risk–reduction eating plan. Many varieties of soups in this chapter are low in fat and feature vitamin-A-rich and vitamin-C-rich vegetables; cruciferous vegetables; lean meats, poultry, and fish; fibrous whole grains; pastas and potatoes; and chemical-free broths and stocks.

If you are a cook with little or no soup-making experience, you will discover that most soups are very simple to prepare. They can easily be made ahead of time in large quantities and frozen in small containers for quick suppers or hot lunches. There is nothing like homemade soup—and once you begin to make your own soups, you will never be able to go back to the packaged or canned variety. The clarity of taste and texture in homemade soup is incomparable.

Beginning with the basics, the foundation of any good soup is the broth (which is also called stock, consommé, or bouillon—these terms are used interchangeably). In this chapter we have included recipes for White Stock (chicken and veal broth), Vegetable Broth, Fish Stock, and Beef Broth.

The success of a good broth depends on the quality and freshness of the ingredients: fresh chicken, meat, and fish; fresh aromatic vegetables like celery, onions, and leeks; and fresh herbs such as parsley, garlic cloves, and bay leaves. To ensure the clarity of the broth, it is vital to adhere to proper cooking temperatures and time (see "Cooking Methods" at the end of this chapter introduction).

All of the broths in this chapter can be served as soups in their original form. Or you can add your own touches—such as chopped scallions, lemon zest, shredded ginger, slivers of lean meat or poultry, fresh parsley, or a sprinkling of grated cheese—for some interesting variations. For example, add thinly sliced mushrooms, slivers of cooked chicken, and the tops of scallions, chopped, to White Stock for a delicately tasty soup. Or add some cooked rice or pasta to the broth and then sprinkle with a bit of parmesan cheese before serving.

Make batches of various broths and freeze them in small containers for future use. Throughout this book different recipes call for very small amounts of broth to moisten a particular dish. A simple way to have a small amount available is to pour homemade broth into ice cube trays. Simply defrost single cubes as needed.

We suggest using the broths listed in this chapter as the bases for our other soups. Canned, commercial broths tend to have a lot of fat, sodium, and chemicals, and some varieties have a somewhat metallic taste.

In this chapter we have tried to include a selection of soups that would satisfy every palate. You'll find some classics like French Onion Soup (mellowed with a touch of brown sugar and baked au gratin with low-fat mozzarella cheese), Gazpacho, Lentil Soup, Vichyssoise (creamy, yet low in fat), and New England Seafood Chowder.

Soups boasting a wealth of vitamin-rich vegetables include Pumpkin Soup in a Shell, Corn Chowder with Tomatoes, Chinese Watercress and Cabbage Soup, Curried Carrot Soup, and Spinach Soup—just to name a few.

There are many soups that are hearty and filling meals in themselves. Some of our entrée soups include Fresh Fish Soup, Vegetable Soup with Pasta, Lamb and Vegetable Soup, and Chicken Chowder. Serve these with a salad and fresh, hot bread.

Bread and soup are a natural combination. The word *soup* is actually derived from the Germanic term *sop*, which meant the bread over which the broth was poured. In some parts of France, *la soupe* still refers to the piece of bread that accompanies the broth or soup. Bread and soup from the earliest times have always been inseparable. In Chapter 7, Pasta, Rice, Grains, and Bread, you will find many varieties of delicious breads that need little or no butter or margarine to taste great. Try Green Chili Corn Bread or Whole-Wheat Biscuits with some of these hearty soups.

Lovers of creamed soups can rejoice—we have wonderfully creamy-tasting soups without the extremely high fat content of the heavy cream bases. Some of these soups include Cream of Brussels Sprouts Soup, Potato and Leek Soup with Carrots, Cream of Broccoli Soup, and Creamy Vegetable Soup. These soups offer a splendid way to begin a special dinner party.

Many of the creamed vegetable soups now available in cans offer about 65% calories from fat. To learn how to make cream bases *without* fat-laden ingredients, try the cooking methods given at the end of this chapter introduction.

If you like Middle Eastern foods, try our Egg-Lemon Soup. Other ethnic soups include Chinese Chicken Noodle Soup, Hot and Sour Soup, Gazpacho, Vegetable Basil Soup, and White Bean and Spinach Soup.

For the creative cook with limited time, there is no end to the kinds of soups you can make simply by searching the refrigerator for leftovers. Start with some White Stock and add leftover vegetables like cauliflower, broccoli, and spinach. Heat on a low flame; add cooked potato to thicken the soup. When heated through (about five minutes), whirl through a blender or food processor. Return to pot and heat a few more minutes. Serve with a sprinkling of parmesan cheese and cracked fresh pepper. This is an "instant" homemade soup, delicious for a chilly evening's meal or a quick and satisfying lunch. Serve with Green Chili Corn Bread.

A wealth of healthful vegetables abound in these soups—like cabbage, broccoli, spinach, brussels sprouts, green peppers, and winter squash—and provide an excellent source of vitamins.

Since the vegetables are cooked and served in the same liquid, no vitamins are thrown down the drain.

All of our soups are lower in fat, so you can have a second cup without feeling guilty. "Soup's on!" won't mean "pounds on" for you from now on.

COOKING METHODS

The success of a good soup depends on the quality of the broth. When making stock or broth, the ingredients should be cooked at a bare simmer. Vegetables, especially, begin to disintegrate when cooked on high heat, and this will make the liquid murky. During the first half hour of cooking, check the broth at frequent intervals to make sure the liquid is not boiling. After the broth is cooked through for flavor, strain the liquid through a mesh strainer or two layers of cheesecloth. This will yield a delicate-tasting and clear stock. Then, if you want a stronger taste, boil the stock down to concentrate the liquid.

To shorten cooking time, meats and vegetables that are chopped into small pieces will yield flavor faster (see Beef Broth). This fast broth will have a lighter flavor because you don't use the bones and trimmings (which make a stronger-tasting stock because of the longer cooking time needed to release their gelatin).

If any fat remains in the broth after straining, chill and then skim the hardened fat from the top. If you are in a hurry, gently skim the top of the broth with a paper towel. If you do have to use packaged or canned broths, do not add any salt to the recipe and remember to chill the can first so that you can easily skim the fat.

Creamed soups, by definition, are a puree of ingredients to which heavy cream has been added—or sometimes a roux of butter and flour—to thicken the soup. Obviously there is no place for heavy cream on a cancer risk–reduction eating plan. But you don't need that kind of cream to get the desired taste and consistency that creamed soups boast. Take a cup of low-fat milk (we use 2% milk throughout the book; skim milk won't work) and mix with 5 tablespoons of nonfat dry milk; you'll have a good cream substitute. It is rich in taste and texture and works wonderfully in the soup base. Adding nonfat dry milk is also a perfect way to add calcium to your diet without adding extra fat.

You can use potato as a base for any creamy vegetable soup.

Pureed potato, or leftover mashed potatoes, work very well as a soup thickener.

A last word on cooking soups: never boil—the ingredients will turn to mush. You want vegetables to be soft, but not over-cooked. The harder or denser the consistency of the vegetable (carrots, turnips, etc.) the longer they will take to cook. If hard vegetables are mixed with soft vegetables like peas or leafy vegetables like spinach, the dense vegetables should be put into the pot first. Then the others should be added according to their consistency.

And remember—soups should always be simmered!

BEEF BROTH

This quickly made broth is a realistic one for people with limited time. The meat and vegetables left after straining can be used for vegetable-beef soup.

> **1 pound boneless beef, all fat removed, cut into small cubes**
> **1½ cups celery, chopped**
> **½ cup carrots, chopped**
> **1 cup leeks, white part only, chopped**
> **½ teaspoon salt**
> **1 quart cold water**

Place all ingredients in a 3-quart pan and bring to a boil, stirring. Partly cover the pan and cook on the lowest possible heat for 1 hour. Strain broth through a mesh strainer. Chill and remove fat from top. Use whenever you need beef broth.

Makes 1 quart/Serves 4

NUTRITIVE VALUES PER SERVING:

FAT	FIBER	VIT. A	VIT. C	CAL	CAL FROM FAT

No analysis is possible for this recipe since the amount of fat in the meat, and the amount of fat removed after the broth has been cooked and chilled vary so much that accurate calculations cannot be made.

CABBAGE SOUP

4 cups water
3 cups unpeeled potatoes, diced
1 cup chopped onion
2 cups chopped carrots
4 cups grated cabbage
½ teaspoon thyme
1 bay leaf
½ teaspoon salt
¼ teaspoon pepper
2 cups low-fat milk
1 15-ounce can tomato sauce

Bring water to boiling in a large pot. Add potatoes, onion, carrots, cabbage, thyme, bay leaf, salt, and pepper. Bring soup to a boil and simmer, uncovered, about 45 minutes or until vegetables are tender. Add milk and tomato sauce and heat gently until soup is heated through.

Serves 8

NUTRITIVE VALUES PER SERVING:

FAT	FIBER	VIT. A	VIT. C	CAL	CAL FROM FAT
1.82gm	5.02gm	9296 IU	41.0mg	136	12%

CHICKEN CHOWDER

3 pounds chicken breasts, boned and skinned
2 bay leaves
1 carrot, coarsely chopped
1 large clove garlic, minced
2 stalks of celery, coarsely chopped
4 sprigs parsley
1 teaspoon salt
$\frac{1}{2}$ teaspoon marjoram
5 cups water
2 tablespoons margarine or butter
1 medium onion, diced
2 carrots, diced
4 medium potatoes, diced
2 cups low-fat milk
$\frac{1}{2}$ cup nonfat dry milk
$\frac{1}{2}$ teaspoon thyme
$\frac{1}{2}$ teaspoon salt
$\frac{1}{4}$ teaspoon pepper
7 cups tomatoes, peeled, seeded, and chopped
    (to peel and seed, see page 224) or 2 28-
    ounce cans, undrained

Rinse chicken and put in large pot with bay leaves, carrot, garlic, celery, parsley, salt, and marjoram. Add water. Bring to a boil, skim off foam, cover, and simmer until chicken is tender, about 1 hour. Remove chicken from pot with a slotted spoon (the liquid and vegetables should remain in the pot). Cut chicken into bite-sized pieces and put aside.

Boil the liquid and vegetables for ½ hour, skimming off any foam or particles. Strain through a mesh strainer. This is your stock.

Melt margarine in another large pot and brown diced onion, carrots, and potato for 5 minutes. Add strained stock, bring to a boil, and simmer 15 minutes or until tender. Combine low-fat milk and dry milk. Add milk, reserved chicken, thyme, salt, pepper, and tomatoes to soup pot. Bring to simmering and simmer 20 minutes. Serve hot.

Serves 10

NUTRITIVE VALUES PER SERVING:

FAT	FIBER	VIT. A	VIT. C	CAL	CAL FROM FAT
7.42gm	7.58gm	4467 IU	56.7mg	339	20%

CHICKEN GUMBO

This hearty soup could serve four as a meal.

1 pound boneless, skinless chicken breast, cut into bite-sized pieces
3 cups water
1 cup chicken broth
1 clove garlic, minced
¼ teaspoon dried red peppers
1 cup onion, chopped
1 bay leaf
⅛ teaspoon sage
¼ teaspoon thyme
2 cups okra, sliced
2 cups tomatoes, chopped
2 cups corn
½ teaspoon salt
¼ teaspoon pepper
2 cups raw brown rice
2 tablespoons margarine or butter
2 tablespoons flour
1 cup chicken broth, additional

Rinse chicken and place in a large soup pot. Cover with water and 1 cup broth and bring to a boil. Skim off foam with a slotted spoon, then add garlic, peppers, onion, bay leaf, sage, and thyme. Cover and simmer for 20 minutes. Skim off any foam.

Add okra, tomatoes, and corn; cover and continue simmering for 20 minutes. Season with salt and pepper.

While soup is simmering, cook rice according to package directions.

In another pan, melt margarine, add flour, and stir over medium heat until golden and bubbly. Add second cup chicken broth, bring to a boil, reduce heat, and whisk until smooth. Add to chicken gumbo and stir to combine and heat through. Serve over hot rice in large soup bowls.

Serves 8

NUTRITIVE VALUES PER SERVING:

FAT	FIBER	VIT. A	VIT. C	CAL	CAL FROM FAT
6.11gm	6.50gm	938 IU	24.4mg	317	17%

CHILLED FRESH TOMATO SOUP

This is a delicious and easy way to use an abundance of fresh tomatoes. Dishes of chopped scallions, cucumber, and avocado may be served as garnishes.

4 pounds tomatoes, peeled and seeded
¼ teaspoon dried basil
2 tablespoons chopped onion
2 cups chicken broth
2 teaspoons sugar
½ teaspoon salt
¼ teaspoon pepper

To peel and seed tomatoes, dip in boiling water for 30 seconds. Immediately place in a bowl of cold water. When cold enough to handle, peel skin off with a knife (it should slip off easily). Cut tomatoes in half (widthwise, not through stem). Squeeze gently to remove seeds.

Cut cores from tomatoes, cut into quarters, and whirl in blender (in 4 batches) until well pureed. Combine with other ingredients in a large bowl, and place in refrigerator for several hours to develop flavor. Serve chilled.

Serves 6

Nutritive Values per Serving:

FAT	FIBER	VIT. A	VIT. C	CAL	CAL FROM FAT
1.00gm	7.25gm	3039 IU	73.1mg	92.4	10%

CHINESE CHICKEN NOODLE SOUP

8 cups chicken broth

½ pound chicken or turkey breast, skinned and boneless, cut in small pieces

4 scallions, sliced

3 carrots, sliced

2 tablespoons soy sauce

1 tablespoon sugar

1 tablespoon sherry

½ teaspoon finely minced fresh ginger

4 ounces whole-wheat vermicelli, broken into 1-inch pieces

Heat broth to boiling in a large soup pot; add all ingredients except vermicelli. Cover and simmer for 20 minutes. Uncover, bring to a boil, add vermicelli, and cook over medium-high heat for 15 minutes. Skim off any foamy particles. Serve hot.

Serves 8

NUTRITIVE VALUES PER SERVING:

FAT	FIBER	VIT. A	VIT. C	CAL	CAL FROM FAT
2.17gm	1.95gm	3319 IU	6.39mg	136	14%

CHINESE WATERCRESS AND CABBAGE SOUP

A terrific soup to serve with an Oriental meal.

¼ cup dried Chinese mushrooms (found in
    Oriental section of market)

1 cup water

3 quarts chicken broth

¼ teaspoon pepper

3 cups watercress, chopped

3 cups cabbage, chopped (curly or Chinese
    cabbage)

¼ cup cornstarch

¼ cup water

¼ cup sherry

2 scallions, sliced

12 ounces tofu (soybean curd), drained and cut
    in small cubes

½ teaspoon salt (optional)

Soak mushrooms in 1 cup water for 30 minutes. Discard any
stems and chop mushrooms, saving the soaking liquid.

Bring broth to a boil in a large soup pot. Add pepper, watercress, and cabbage. Simmer 3 minutes. Stir cornstarch and ¼
cup water together and add to soup. Bring to a boil, stirring
constantly, and simmer 1 minute. Stir in mushrooms and soaking liquid, sherry, scallions, and tofu. Taste and add salt, if
necessary. Heat thoroughly, but don't boil. Serve hot.

Serves 12

NUTRITIVE VALUES PER SERVING:

FAT	FIBER	VIT. A	VIT. C	CAL	CAL FROM FAT
2.37gm	.97	349 IU	13.2mg	63.8	33%

CORN CHOWDER WITH TOMATOES

2 tablespoons vegetable or chicken broth
½ cup chopped onion
1 cup grated carrots
3 cups corn
1 cup chopped tomatoes
3 cups water
½ teaspoon salt
¼ teaspoon pepper
1 tablespoon margarine or butter
1 tablespoon flour
1½ cups low-fat milk
1 ounce grated part-skim mozzarella cheese
2 tablespoons diced mild green chilies (canned)

Heat broth in a large saucepan. Add onions and carrots and soften for 5 minutes. Add corn, tomatoes, water, salt, and pepper. Bring to a boil and simmer for 30 minutes.

Melt margarine in another saucepan and blend in flour. Cook, stirring, over low heat until golden brown. Add milk, bring to a boil, reduce heat, and whisk together until smooth and thickened. Add to soup. Stir in cheese and chilies and heat thoroughly over low heat. Serve hot.

Serves 6

NUTRITIVE VALUES PER SERVING:

FAT	FIBER	VIT. A	VIT. C	CAL	CAL FROM FAT
4.54gm	6.87gm	3624 IU	18.5mg	154	27%

CREAM OF BROCCOLI SOUP

3 cups broccoli florets and peeled stems, finely
   chopped
1½ cups water
1 tablespoon margarine
½ cup chopped onions
1 tablespoon flour
3 cups low-fat milk
½ teaspoon salt
½ teaspoon pepper
¼ teaspoon paprika
⅛ teaspoon cayenne pepper
¼ teaspoon celery seed

Place broccoli florets and stems in a 3-quart saucepan; add 1½
cups water and bring to a boil. Simmer, covered, 10 minutes.
Drain, reserving the liquid.

Melt margarine in a larger saucepan; sauté onion until soft.
Blend in flour and cook until thickened. Add milk, broccoli, salt,
pepper, paprika, cayenne pepper, and celery seed. Blend together and heat slowly. Serve hot.

Serves 6

NUTRITIVE VALUES PER SERVING:

FAT	FIBER	VIT. A	VIT. C	CAL	CAL FROM FAT
3.32gm	5.05gm	2219 IU	72.4mg	101	29%

CREAM OF
BRUSSELS SPROUTS SOUP

1½ pounds fresh brussels sprouts

2 scallions, sliced

1½ cups diced unpeeled potato

2 teaspoons margarine or butter

¼ teaspoon celery seed

½ teaspoon salt

¼ teaspoon pepper

5 cups chicken stock

2 egg yolks

1 cup low-fat milk

5 tablespoons nonfat dry milk

Remove stem from each brussels sprout. Cut an *X* in root of each sprout; place in saucepan and steam until done (about 20 minutes). If roots are still hard after cooking, remove with a paring knife.

In a large pot, sauté scallions and potato in margarine for 5 minutes. Add sprouts, celery seed, salt, pepper, and stock to the cooked scallion mixture. Simmer about 30 minutes, then puree until smooth. Whisk eggs, low-fat milk, and dry milk together. Add milk mixture to soup, whisking constantly, and simmer gently until thoroughly heated. Serve hot.

Serves 6

NUTRITIVE VALUES PER SERVING:

FAT	FIBER	VIT. A	VIT. C	CAL	CAL FROM FAT
5.58qm	4.89gm	5010 IU	111mg	171	29%

CREAMY VEGETABLE SOUP

1½ tablespoons margarine or butter
1 pound broccoli florets and peeled stems,
    chopped
1 pound zucchini, sliced
12 cups broth
1 bunch parsley, chopped
1 bunch watercress, chopped
½ teaspoon salt
¼ teaspoon pepper
1½ cups low-fat yogurt

Melt margarine in a large pot; sauté broccoli until softened. Add zucchini and cook 5 minutes more. Add broth, parsley, watercress, salt, and pepper. Simmer for 20 minutes, uncovered.

Puree until smooth. Add yogurt and heat gently, whisking to combine. May be served hot or chilled.

Serves 10

NUTRITIVE VALUES PER SERVING:

FAT	FIBER	VIT. A	VIT. C	CAL	CAL FROM FAT
3.89gm	4.70gm	3714 IU	57.8mg	91.8	38%*

*Because the fat content of this soup is higher than recommended, lower the amount of fat in the rest of your meal.

CURRIED CARROT SOUP

1 cup chopped onions
4 cups chopped carrots
1 tablespoon margarine or butter
½ teaspoon curry powder
½ teaspoon ground cumin
½ teaspoon ground coriander
½ teaspoon salt
¼ teaspoon white pepper
5 cups water
1 cup low-fat cottage cheese
1 cup low-fat milk
1 teaspoon fresh lemon juice
½ cup chopped green bell pepper
½ cup chopped parsley

In a large pot, sauté onion and carrots in margarine for 5 minutes; season with curry, cumin, and coriander while sautéing. Add salt, pepper, and water and simmer, partially covered, for 15 minutes. Transfer to blender and puree. Return to pot.

Mix cottage cheese, milk, and lemon juice in blender until very smooth and stir into soup. Heat through on low heat. Garnish each serving with green bell pepper and parsley. May be served hot or chilled.

Serves 6

NUTRITIVE VALUES PER SERVING:

FAT	FIBER	VIT. A	VIT. C	CAL	CAL FROM FAT
3.73gm	5.63gm	11,524 IU	33.8mg	111	30%

EGG-LEMON SOUP

6 cups chicken broth

½ cup raw brown rice

2 eggs

3 tablespoons fresh lemon juice

2 tablespoons cornstarch

2 tablespoons water

¼ teaspoon salt (optional)

Bring broth to a boil in a 3-quart saucepan; add rice. Reduce heat to low, cover, and simmer 35 minutes. Beat eggs with whisk and beat in lemon juice. Whisk ½ cup of hot stock into eggs. Slowly add egg mixture back into soup, whisking constantly. Mix cornstarch with 2 tablespoons water and add to soup, stirring constantly. Bring soup to a boil, reduce heat, and simmer 5 minutes, stirring often. Taste and add salt, if necessary. Serve hot.

Serves 6

NUTRITIVE VALUES PER SERVING:

FAT	FIBER	VIT. A	VIT. C	CAL	CAL FROM FAT
3.37gm	1.19gm	128 IU	3.6mg	117	26%

FISH STOCK

**2 pounds fish bones and trimmings (including 6
    ounces white fish flesh)**
1 onion, chopped
1 garlic clove, peeled and cut in half
1 carrot, coarsely chopped
2 celery stalks, coarsely chopped
1 cup white wine
½ cup parsley sprigs
2 bay leaves
3 whole peppercorns
¼ teaspoon thyme
2 quarts water

Place all ingredients in a stock pot and bring to a boil. Skim off
any foam from the top. Partially cover and simmer for 2 hours.
Strain and refrigerate; remove any fat that rises to the top. Use
whenever you need fish stock or broth.

Makes about 5 cups/Serves 5

Nutritive Values per Serving:

FAT	FIBER	VIT. A	VIT. C	CAL	CAL FROM FAT
.47gm	0	2189 IU	15.6mg	73	6%

FRENCH ONION SOUP

2 tablespoons margarine or butter
1½ pounds onions, quartered and thinly sliced
2 cups grated carrots
1 tablespoon brown sugar
1 teaspoon paprika
3 tablespoons flour
6 cups beef broth
½ teaspoon thyme
¼ teaspoon salt (or none if using canned broth)
¼ teaspoon pepper
6 toasted whole-wheat croutons (1–1½ ounces each)
⅓ cup grated part-skim mozzarella cheese
2 tablespoons parmesan cheese, freshly grated

Heat margarine in a soup pot. Add onions and carrots and cook, covered, over very low heat for 20 minutes. Remove lid and add brown sugar. Stir until onions are browned. Stir in paprika and flour and stir to coat onions. Add broth, thyme, salt, and pepper. Simmer, uncovered, over low heat for 30 minutes.

While soup is simmering, prepare croutons. Dry slices of whole-wheat french bread (or white french bread if whole-wheat is unavailable) in a 250°F oven for 30 minutes.

Ladle soup into ovenproof soup bowls. Place on baking sheet. Put a crouton into each bowl and sprinkle with cheeses. Place 4 inches below broiler and broil for 3–4 minutes, until the cheese is bubbling and slightly browned.

If you don't have individual soup bowls that are ovenproof, heat soup piping hot, dish into bowls, place the crouton and cheeses on top of the soup, and serve immediately.

Serves 6

NUTRITIVE VALUES PER SERVING:

FAT	FIBER	VIT. A	VIT. C	CAL	CAL FROM FAT
7.66gm	5.65gm	5665 IU	11.1mg	233	30%

FRESH FISH SOUP

2 tablespoons margarine or butter
4 medium potatoes, thinly sliced
2 medium onions, thinly sliced
½ teaspoon salt
¼ teaspoon pepper
⅛ teaspoon ground allspice
¼ teaspoon thyme
1½ pounds boneless fish fillets (any
    combination of fish)
2 cups low-fat milk

Melt margarine in bottom of large soup pot. Remove from heat. Arrange half the potatoes in bottom of pan. Cover with half the onions. Combine salt, pepper, allspice, and thyme. Sprinkle ⅓ of spice mixture over onions.

Add all the fish fillets; sprinkle with ⅓ of spice mixture. Add remaining potatoes, top with remaining onions, and sprinkle with remaining ⅓ of spices. Gently cover with water (to barely cover mixture).

Cover pan and place on stove over lowest heat for 2 hours, or until potatoes are tender. Add milk after soup has cooked 2 hours. Stir gently but thoroughly to combine all flavors, and cook for an additional hour. Serve hot.

Serves 8

NUTRITIVE VALUES PER SERVING:

FAT	FIBER	VIT. A	VIT. C	CAL	CAL FROM FAT
5.08gm	2.65gm	249 IU	18.5mg	197	23%

GAZPACHO

8 cups chicken broth

4 cups tomato juice

3 cloves garlic, minced

1 tablespoon olive oil

2 tablespoons red wine vinegar

Few drops tabasco sauce (hot pepper sauce)

1 teaspoon worcestershire sauce

½ teaspoon salt

¼ teaspoon pepper

¼ head celery, diced

2 cucumbers, diced

2 red or green bell peppers, diced

½ medium onion, diced

2 large tomatoes, peeled, seeded, and diced (to
   peel and seed, see page 224)

¼ cup chopped chives

Place broth and tomato juice in a large bowl or pan. Puree garlic and oil in a blender. Add red wine vinegar, tabasco, worcestershire, salt, and pepper and blend. Add to broth and juice. Stir celery, cucumbers, peppers, onions, and tomatoes into broth and juice. Chill for several hours. Serve in chilled bowls, sprinkling each serving with chives.

Serves 12

NUTRITIVE VALUES PER SERVING:

FAT	FIBER	VIT. A	VIT. C	CAL	CAL FROM FAT
2.09gm	1.95gm	1050 IU	45.0mg	53.6	35%*

*Because the fat content of this soup is higher than recommended, lower the amount of fat in the rest of your meal.

HOT AND SOUR SOUP

The "hot" comes from the pepper, and the "sour" from the vinegar. The more you add the spicier and more piquant the soup will be. If you tend to like mild foods, you might want to start with less than the suggested minimum amount.

¼ cup dried **Chinese mushrooms** (found in Oriental section of market)

½ cup **bean threads** (found in Oriental section of market)

6 cups **chicken broth**

4 ounces shredded cooked **chicken breast**

½ cup grated **carrots**

¼ cup sliced **scallions**

½ cup sliced **water chestnuts**

1 teaspoon **soy sauce**

1 teaspoon **sugar**

3-4 tablespoons **red wine vinegar**

½-¾ teaspoons **black pepper**

2 tablespoons **cornstarch**

2 tablespoons **water**

1 **egg**, beaten

1 teaspoon **sesame oil** (found in Oriental section of market)

8 ounces **tofu** (soybean curd), cubed

½ cup fresh **cilantro** (coriander) optional

Soak mushrooms and bean threads, separately, in water to cover for 30 minutes. Drain, discarding tough stems from mushrooms.

Simmer chicken broth with chicken, mushrooms, bean threads, carrots, scallions, and water chestnuts for 10 minutes. Still simmering, add soy sauce, sugar, 3 tablespoons vinegar, and ½ teaspoon pepper and stir. Mix cornstarch and water together. Heat soup to boiling and add cornstarch-water mixture. Reduce heat and stir until soup is slightly thickened.

Off heat, stir in beaten egg. Add sesame oil and tofu and gently heat through. Taste for flavors; add more vinegar or pepper as needed. Serve hot.

May be sprinkled with fresh cilantro just before serving.

Serves 6–8

NUTRITIVE VALUES PER SERVING:

FAT	FIBER	VIT. A	VIT. C	CAL	CAL FROM FAT
3.34gm	1.35gm	1147 IU	2.77mg	81.2	37%*

*Because the fat content of this soup is higher than recommended, lower the amount of fat in the rest of your meal.

LAMB AND VEGETABLE SOUP

1½ pounds boneless, lean lamb, cut in 1-inch
    cubes

2 tablespoons olive oil

1 cup sliced onion

6 carrots, sliced into bite-sized pieces

12 small whole boiling onions, peeled and
    halved

2 tablespoons flour

6 cups chicken stock

1 cup water

12 small new potatoes, cut in quarters

1½ cups diced rutabagas or turnips

3 bay leaves

2 garlic cloves, minced

1 teaspoon fennel seeds

½ teaspoon salt

½ teaspoon pepper

3 large romaine lettuce leaves, coarsely chopped

1½ cups asparagus tips, fresh or frozen, cut into
    1-inch pieces

1½ cups artichoke hearts, canned or frozen,
    sliced

1 cup finely chopped parsley

Trim lamb of all fat. In a large skillet, sauté lamb in oil over medium heat until well browned. With a slotted spoon, transfer lamb to an ovenproof casserole dish. Add sliced onion, carrots, and boiling onions to skillet and cook until lightly browned. Add carrots and boiling onions to casserole with the lamb, leaving sliced onions in skillet. Blend flour into onions in skillet, stirring to coat onions with the flour. Add stock and water and bring to a boil. Reduce heat and simmer 5 minutes, whisking until thickened.

Pour mixture through a mesh sieve into the casserole containing the lamb and vegetables, pressing on onions to extract all juices into the casserole. Add new potatoes, rutabagas, bay leaves, garlic, fennel, salt, pepper, and lettuce to the casserole and stir to combine all ingredients. Cover and bake at 375°F for 1 hour, or simmer on top of your stove over low heat, covered, for about 1½ hours.

Add asparagus and artichoke hearts to the soup, stir, and cook 30 minutes more—at 300°F in the oven, or on very low heat on the stove. Garnish with finely chopped parsley just before serving.

Serves 12 as a soup, or 8 as an entrée

NUTRITIVE VALUES PER SERVING:

FAT	FIBER	VIT. A	VIT. C	CAL	CAL FROM FAT
11.2gm	12.1gm	6614 IU	47.8mg	358	28%

LENTIL SOUP

2 tablespoons olive oil
2 cups lentils
1 cup chopped onion
1 cup chopped carrots
¼ cup chopped parsley
2 cloves garlic, minced
¾ teaspoon salt
½ teaspoon pepper
½ teaspoon thyme
8 cups water
2 cups chopped tomatoes
2 tablespoons white or red wine vinegar

Heat olive oil in a soup pot and sauté lentils, onion, carrots, parsley, garlic, salt, pepper, and thyme for 15 minutes over medium heat. Add water and tomatoes and simmer, covered, for 1½ hours. Add vinegar and simmer 30 minutes longer. Serve hot.

Serves 10

NUTRITIVE VALUES PER SERVING:

FAT	FIBER	VIT. A	VIT. C	CAL	CAL FROM FAT
3.27gm	6.74gm	2263 IU	19.1mg	170	17%

NEW ENGLAND
SEAFOOD CHOWDER

1½ cups whole-wheat croutons, using 4 slices of
    bread

3 tablespoons margarine or butter

4 cups sliced onions

3 tablespoons flour

2 cups clam juice

2 cups water

5 cups sliced potatoes

1 teaspoon thyme

¾ teaspoon salt

½ teaspoon pepper

2 pounds boneless fish fillets, cut into bite-sized
    chunks

2 cups low-fat milk

½ cup chopped parsley

To prepare croutons, cube 4 slices whole-wheat bread (or white,
if whole-wheat is not available). Dry cubes on baking sheet in a
250°F oven for 30 minutes.

While croutons are baking, prepare soup. Heat margarine in a
large pot and sauté onions for 10 minutes. Stir in flour and cook
2 minutes, blending well. Add clam juice and water and bring to
a boil. Reduce heat and stir until thickened.

Add potatoes, thyme, salt, and pepper and simmer for 10
minutes. Add fish and milk to the soup and continue to simmer
for about 5 minutes, or until fish is just cooked (opaque rather
than translucent). Don't overcook. Serve hot, sprinkled with
parsley and croutons.

Serves 12 as a soup, or 8 as an entrée

NUTRITIVE VALUES PER SERVING:

FAT	FIBER	VIT. A	VIT. C	CAL	CAL FROM FAT
4.96gm	3.42gm	426 IU	18.8mg	198	23%

POTATO AND LEEK SOUP WITH CARROTS

3 tablespoons oil
3 tablespoons margarine or butter
4 cups washed leeks, sliced
4 pounds unpeeled potatoes, chopped *8 med, potatoes*
2 small rutabagas or turnips, chopped (set aside
  ¼ cup for garnish)
1 pound carrots, chopped (set aside ¼ cup for
  garnish) *41g. or 6 small*
3 quarts chicken or vegetable stock
1 teaspoon salt
½ teaspoon white pepper
1 cup low-fat milk
¾ cup chopped parsley

In a large pot, melt oil and margarine and sauté leeks for 10 minutes over low heat (don't brown). Add potatoes, rutabagas, carrots, stock, salt, and pepper and simmer, partially covered, for 45 minutes. Puree slightly, leaving some texture. Return puree to pot; add milk and simmer gently until thoroughly heated.

Serve hot, garnishing each portion with a sprinkling of parsley and some of the reserved carrots and rutabagas.

Serves 12

NUTRITIVE VALUES PER SERVING:

FAT	FIBER	VIT. A	VIT. C	CAL	CAL FROM FAT
8.17gm	8.20gm	4768 IU	47.9	254	29%

PUMPKIN SOUP IN A SHELL

This soup may be served in a bowl, but the pumpkin shell is festive and very attractive.

> **1 pumpkin, about 6 pounds**
> **6 cups chicken broth**
> **1 cup thinly sliced onion**
> **1 clove garlic, minced**
> **½ teaspoon thyme**
> **¼ teaspoon pepper**
> **1 cup low-fat milk**
> **¼-½ teaspoon salt (optional—or none if using canned broth)**
> **1 cup finely chopped parsley**

Cut top off pumpkin and scoop out seeds. Cut out enough of the pumpkin meat to make 2½ cups of diced pumpkin cubes. Be careful not to cut into the shell, if you intend to use it as a serving bowl.

Bring broth to a boil in a large pot. Add onion, garlic, thyme, pepper, and pumpkin cubes, and bring to a second boil. Reduce heat and simmer, uncovered, for 40 minutes.

Puree soup in blender or processor and return to pot. Bring to a boil, reduce heat to simmer, and add milk. Taste and add salt (only if necessary). Simmer for 10 more minutes, until soup is very hot. Immediately pour into pumpkin shell.

Bring soup-filled pumpkin shell to table, and dish up each portion from shell. Garnish each serving with parsley as soup is dished up.

Serves 8

NUTRITIVE VALUES PER SERVING:

FAT	FIBER	VIT. A	VIT. C	CAL	CAL FROM FAT
1.72gm	2.45gm	5634 IU	18.8mg	65.8	24%

SPINACH SOUP

2 cups low-fat milk

5 cups chicken broth

2 packages frozen chopped spinach, defrosted
but not drained

1 teaspoon worcestershire sauce

½ teaspoon salt (or none if using canned broth)

¼ teaspoon pepper

1 tablespoon margarine or butter

1 tablespoon flour

Bring milk and broth to a boil in a large pot. Stir in spinach, worcestershire, salt (if used), and pepper. Bring to a second boil, lower heat, and simmer 15 minutes, partially covered.

While soup is simmering, make a roux: melt margarine over medium heat, add flour, and cook, stirring constantly, until golden brown. Remove from heat.

After soup has simmered for 15 minutes, reheat the roux over medium heat, add 1 cup soup into the roux, whisk to combine, and add back into the soup. Blend well and heat 5 more minutes. Serve hot.

Serves 8

NUTRITIVE VALUES PER SERVING:

FAT	FIBER	VIT. A	VIT. C	CAL	CAL FROM FAT
3.56gm	4.55gm	6370 IU	15.4mg	81.4	39%*

*Because the fat content of this soup is higher than recommended, lower the amount of fat in the rest of your meal.

TOMATO BOUILLON

This bouillon is a wonderful first course for an elegant dinner.

3 1-pound cans tomatoes, undrained
1 cup chopped turnips
2 carrots, chopped
½ green bell pepper, chopped
1 cup chopped onion
4 peppercorns
¼ teaspoon salt
½ teaspoon thyme
½ teaspoon sugar
¼ cup port wine
1 tablespoon fresh lemon juice
6 tablespoons chopped parsley

Put tomatoes, undrained, into a large pot, breaking them up with a fork. Add turnips, carrots, green pepper, and onion to the pot. Season with peppercorns, salt, thyme, and sugar. Cover pot tightly and bring to a boil. Lower heat and simmer for one hour, stirring once or twice. Cool and strain the soup through a mesh sieve, pressing the juices out of the vegetables and into the bouillon. Return the bouillon to a clean pan and add the port and lemon juice. Bring to a boil, reduce heat, and simmer 5 minutes. Serve hot, sprinkling each serving with 1 tablespoon parsley.

Serves 6

NUTRITIVE VALUES PER SERVING:

FAT	FIBER	VIT. A	VIT. C	CAL	CAL FROM FAT
.34gm	0	3736 IU	44.4mg	51.5	6%

TOMATO SOUP

1 tablespoon margarine
3 medium carrots, minced
1 stalk celery, minced
2 medium onions, minced
10 large tomatoes, peeled, seeded, and chopped
(to peel and seed, see page 224)
½ teaspoon sugar
½ teaspoon basil
½ teaspoon thyme
½ teaspoon salt
¼ teaspoon pepper
3 tablespoons freshly grated parmesan cheese
3 tablespoons chopped parsley

Heat margarine in a large soup pot. Sauté carrots, celery, and onions over medium-low heat for 20 minutes, or until soft. Don't brown. Add tomatoes, sugar, basil, thyme, salt, and pepper to the pot and cook 30 minutes. Soup may be pureed at this point, if desired. Serve piping hot, sprinkling each serving with 1½ teaspoons parmesan and 1½ teaspoons parsley.

Serves 6

NUTRITIVE VALUES PER SERVING:

FAT	FIBER	VIT. A	VIT. C	CAL	CAL FROM FAT
3.12gm	6.57gm	6172 IU	57.1mg	99	28%

VEGETABLE BASIL SOUP

3 quarts chicken stock

1 pound cauliflower, chopped

½ pound green beans, sliced

1 cup chopped onion

2 pounds new potatoes, chopped

2 pounds carrots, sliced

6 tomatoes, peeled, seeded, and chopped (to
    peel and seed, see page 224)

¼ cup Spinach Pesto (see Index*)

Bring stock to a boil. Add vegetables, bring to second boil, and simmer, partially covered, for 1 hour. Add Spinach Pesto and blend well. Heat thoroughly before serving.

*Commercial pesto is available in either the fine food or freezer section of your market. However, we highly recommend the Spinach Pesto from this book. It is quick to make, lower in fat, and absolutely delicious.

Serves 12

NUTRITIVE VALUES PER SERVING:

FAT	FIBER	VIT. A	VIT. C	CAL	CAL FROM FAT
2.91gm	8.67gm	9225 IU	60.9mg	159	16%

VEGETABLE BROTH

3 cups carrots, coarsely chopped
1 bunch parsley, coarsely chopped
3 cups celery, coarsely chopped
4 cloves garlic, quartered
2 onions, chopped
3 bay leaves
½ teaspoon sage
½ teaspoon thyme
1 teaspoon salt
¼ teaspoon white pepper
2 quarts cold water
2 tablespoons fresh lemon juice

Place all ingredients in a large pot; bring to a boil. Reduce heat, cover, and simmer for 1 hour.

Cool and strain through a mesh strainer, pressing juice out of vegetables. Discard vegetables. Store broth in refrigerator or freeze.

Makes about 2 quarts

NUTRITIVE VALUES PER SERVING:

FAT	FIBER	VIT. A	VIT. C	CAL	CAL FROM FAT
.32gm	6.64gm	7533 IU	36.1mg	35.5	8%

VEGETABLE SOUP WITH PASTA

Add cooked chicken or turkey for a "full meal" soup.

2 cups chopped onions
3 tablespoons olive oil
2 cloves garlic, minced
1 large green or red bell pepper, chopped
1 pound carrots, sliced
2 cups chopped unpeeled potatoes
2 cups chopped turnips
10 cups chicken broth
2 pounds green beans, sliced into small pieces
2 cups cooked whole-wheat pasta shells (small size)
½ teaspoon salt
¼ teaspoon pepper
1½ cups chopped parsley

In a large pot, sauté onions in oil until soft. Add garlic, bell pepper, and carrots. Cook 5 minutes. Add potatoes, turnips, and broth and simmer, partially covered, about 10 minutes, until potatoes and turnips are almost tender. Add green beans and simmer 5 minutes. Add cooked pasta, salt, and pepper and simmer 10 minutes. Serve hot, sprinkling each serving with 2 tablespoons parsley.

Serves 12

NUTRITIVE VALUES PER SERVING:

FAT	FIBER	VIT. A	VIT. C	CAL	CAL FROM FAT
7.88gm	4.84gm	5285 IU	50.5mg	152	29%

VICHYSSOISE

6 cups chicken broth
4 cups sliced peeled potatoes
3 cups sliced leeks (white part only)
½ teaspoon salt (or none if using canned broth)
¼ teaspoon white pepper
1 cup low-fat milk
5 tablespoons nonfat dry milk
¼ cup finely chopped chives
¼ cup finely chopped watercress

Place broth in a large pot and bring to a boil. Reduce heat, add potatoes and leeks, and simmer for 30 minutes, until vegetables are tender.

Puree soup until smooth in a blender or processor. Transfer to a large bowl or pan. Stir in salt, pepper, low-fat milk, and dry milk. Mix well with a whisk and chill.

Serve in chilled soup cups; sprinkle each serving with ½ tablespoon chives and ½ tablespoon watercress.

Serves 8

NUTRITIVE VALUES PER SERVING:

FAT	FIBER	VIT. A	VIT. C	CAL	CAL FROM FAT
1.66gm	3.68mg	196 IU	22.0mg	122	12%

WHITE BEAN AND SPINACH SOUP

1 pound white beans
4 cups water for soaking
4 cups fresh water
8 cups beef broth
1½ cups chopped onions
2 cups grated carrots
⅛ teaspoon cayenne pepper
¼ teaspoon black pepper
½ teaspoon thyme
4 cloves garlic, minced
3 bay leaves
6 cups fresh spinach leaves, torn into pieces
2 16-ounce cans tomatoes, drained and coarsely
    chopped (reserve liquid)
½ teaspoon sugar
½ teaspoon salt (or none if using canned broth)

Soak beans overnight in 4 cups water. Drain off soaking water;
cover beans with 4 cups fresh water. Add beef broth and bring to
a boil. Reduce heat and add onion, carrots, cayenne, black
pepper, thyme, garlic, and bay leaves. Bring to a second boil,
reduce heat, and simmer until beans are tender (about 1 hour).

When beans are completely tender, add spinach leaves, tomatoes and their reserved liquid, sugar, and salt and bring to a boil.
Reduce heat, simmer for 5 minutes, and serve hot.

Serves 8

NUTRITIVE VALUES PER SERVING:

1.58gm	8.62gm	8443 IU	45.6mg	257	6%

WHITE STOCK

2 pounds veal bones
3 pounds chicken bones (or wings, necks, backs)
3 quarts cold water
1½ cups chopped carrots
3 cups sliced leeks
1 cup chopped celery
½ cup parsley sprigs
3 bay leaves
6 peppercorns
½ teaspoon marjoram
2 garlic cloves, cut in half

Rinse veal and chicken bones under running water. Place veal and chicken bones in a stock pot and add 3 quarts cold water. Bring to a boil and skim off foam.

Add carrots, leeks, celery, parsley, bay leaves, peppercorns, marjoram, and garlic. Bring to a second boil and reduce heat. Partially cover pot, lower heat, and simmer 3–4 hours. Strain through a mesh sieve and refrigerate. When chilled, skim off any fat that rises to the top.

May be used whenever you need white stock, chicken stock, or chicken broth.

Makes 2 quarts/Serves 8

NUTRITIVE VALUES PER SERVING:

FAT	FIBER	VIT. A	VIT. C	CAL	CAL FROM FAT
.22gm	0	3435 IU	14.6mg	19.3	10%

3
Salads

Black-Eyed Peas Vinaigrette
Carrot and Orange Salad
Chinese Noodle Salad with
  Peanut Sauce
Coleslaw Dijon
Dilled Carrots
French Potato Salad
Iced Summer Fruit Salad
Lemon-Broccoli Salad
Lentil Salad with Feta Cheese
Marinated Black Bean Salad
Mexican Chicken Salad
Molded Gazpacho Salad
Oriental Turkey Salad with Cilantro
Papaya and Cucumber Salad

Pasta and Broccoli Salad
Pasta Salad with Fresh Tomatoes
Rice Salad
Rice-Stuffed Tomatoes
Salade Niçoise
Shredded Chicken Salad
Spinach and Grapefruit Salad
Spinach Salad Supreme
Summer Salad
Taco Salad
Tangy Carrot Salad
Tomato and Watercress Salad
Vegetable Salad
White Bean Salad

Salads

A well-planned salad can be the perfect course. It is quick and simple to prepare, contains varied textures and tastes, looks fresh and appealing, and—most important—fills many requirements of a cancer risk–reduction eating plan. The best salads are high in vitamins A and C, low in fat, and contain a substantial amount of dietary fiber. Make delicious and nutritious combinations from fresh leafy greens; cruciferous vegetables; vitamin-C-rich fruits; vegetables high in beta-carotene; high-fiber legumes and beans; lean meats, fish, and poultry; part-skim cheeses; rice; pasta; and fresh herbs.

Salads are *not* just for dinner! Begin breakfast or brunch with a fresh fruit compote like Iced Summer Fruit Salad instead of a glass of juice. If you use fruits like apples, peaches, or nectarines in the salad, sprinkle with a little fresh lemon juice to prevent discoloration (which happens almost immediately). For the maximum intake of vitamins and fiber, leave the skin on all soft fruits whenever possible. And when using grapefruits and oranges, use the *whole* fruit—fiber is not only in the flesh of the fruit itself but also in the white skin and the translucent membranes separating the selections. The amounts may be minimal, but they add up—whenever possible, use *every part* of fruits and vegetables in food preparation.

Eat a fresh vegetable or leafy green salad of your creation at both lunch and dinner. For something a little unusual, try Spinach and Grapefruit Salad, Papaya and Cucumber Salad, or Lemon-Broccoli Salad.

Since "salad" means "lettuce" to many people, remember this basic rule when preparing salads: the darker and more colorful the lettuce leaf, the more vitamins it contains. Experiment with chicory, escarole, tangy and pungent mustard greens (you only need a few), spinach, watercress, and carrot tops. To add vitamins to a pale Belgian endive or iceberg salad, mix with a darker lettuce like watercress and add a ripe tomato (otherwise, you are basically eating dressing).

Never soak lettuce; you will lose some of the water-soluble vitamins to the water. Just rinse leafy greens with cool water, and pat dry or spin dry in a salad spinner. Store whole leaves in the refrigerator in an airtight plastic bag or container. When you are ready to serve the salad, tear or cut the greens into bite-size pieces. Then add other vegetables like tomatoes, carrots, peppers, etc., cutting them up at the last minute so they don't wilt or dry out.

A salad of crisp greens, fresh vegetables, and a good dressing is a fine addition to any meal, but don't stop there: raid your refrigerator for hearty, healthful additions. Cold brown rice with its crunchy texture is delicious in a salad, and also adds vitamins and fiber. The same is true for garbanzos, peas, lima beans, and kidney beans. Often called "magic beans," these different legumes are chewy and satisfying, fill you up, and are low in fat, especially compared to a serving of meat. And just a ½-cup cooked portion will add 5–10 grams of fiber to your meal. (To store canned kidney beans, rinse thoroughly after opening. Otherwise, the thick packing liquid becomes rancid within a couple of days.)

Add last night's al dente steamed vegetables like cauliflower and broccoli. Save leftover spaghetti, ziti, shells, and other pasta for a hearty Pasta Salad (see Index), or as an addition to a mixed green salad.

This chapter offers some interesting and flavorful dishes: try Marinated Black Bean Salad in the winter months when many fresh vegetables are unavailable, Molded Gazpacho Salad at a buffet supper, or Carrot and Orange Salad when the entrée calls for a salad with a touch of sweetness.

Summer is the perfect time for salad: no meal could be more satisfying on a steamy summer night than Oriental Turkey Salad with Cilantro, Salade Niçoise, or Taco Salad. Or for a light lunch on the patio, serve Lentil Salad with Feta Cheese, Shredded Chicken Salad, or Pasta Salad with Fresh Tomatoes.

Calorie counters will appreciate Rice-Stuffed Tomatoes, Vegetable Salad, and Pasta and Broccoli Salad among others in this chapter.

Any salad is incomplete without the right dressing. Chapter 8, Sauces and Salad Dressings, suggests many delicious dressings, from piquant Soy-Sesame Vinaigrette to delicate Raspberry Vinegar Dressing.

Become known as the "salad person" and your expertise will be sought out for picnics and all kinds of parties. And who will ever guess that your delicious salads also provide such a wealth of healthful foods!

BLACK-EYED PEAS VINAIGRETTE

Particularly good with a sausage entrée.

SALAD

1 pound black-eyed peas
1 cup grated carrots
1 cup chopped onions
1 cup chopped parsley

DRESSING

¼ cup vegetable or chicken broth, fat removed
2 tablespoons olive oil
¼ cup red wine vinegar
2 cloves garlic, minced
1 tablespoon oregano
1½ teaspoons dijon mustard
½ teaspoon pepper
1 teaspoon salt

Cook black-eyed peas according to package directions. Mix dressing ingredients together while peas are cooking. When peas are done, drain well. Toss with carrots, onions, and parsley. Add dressing and gently toss. Cover; refrigerate and marinate several hours or overnight before serving.

Serves 12

CARROT AND ORANGE SALAD

This refreshing salad is especially good with poultry or anything spicy.

SALAD

4 carrots, grated
2 oranges, sectioned
2 cups chopped watercress

DRESSING

1 tablespoon olive oil
1 tablespoon honey
1½ teaspoons dijon mustard
3 tablespoons white wine vinegar
3 tablespoons orange juice
¼ teaspoon salt

Cover grated carrots with boiling water and let set for 5 minutes. Drain well (save liquid for soup), pressing liquid from carrots. Let carrots cool a bit. Cut oranges into bite-sized pieces. Wash and dry watercress and remove the tough stems.

Mix dressing ingredients together and toss with carrots, oranges, and watercress. Marinate for at least two hours before serving.

Serves 6

CHINESE NOODLE SALAD WITH PEANUT SAUCE

SALAD

¼ cup toasted sesame seeds

½ pound whole-wheat vermicelli (white may be substituted)

2 cups cooked turkey, cut in small cubes

2 scallions, sliced

SAUCE

3 tablespoons rice wine vinegar or white wine vinegar

2 tablespoons peanut butter

1 tablespoon honey

1 tablespoon dijon mustard

2 tablespoons soy sauce

1½ teaspoons hot chili oil (found in Oriental section of market)

2 tablespoons Chinese sesame oil (found in Oriental section of market)

3 tablespoons fresh orange juice

To toast sesame seeds, heat for 5 minutes in an ungreased frying pan on medium heat, tossing frequently, until golden brown.

Cook vermicelli according to package directions. Rinse under cold water. Drain well.

Mix sauce ingredients together in blender. Toss turkey with sauce in a large bowl. Toss in vermicelli, in batches, until all ingredients are well combined. Pour onto serving platter and sprinkle with sesame seeds and scallions.

Serves 10 as a salad or 6 as an entrée

NUTRITIVE VALUES PER SERVING:

FAT	FIBER	VIT. A	VIT. C	CAL	CAL FROM FAT
6.62gm	2.89gm	10.4 IU	3.01mg	202	29%

COLESLAW DIJON

SLAW

6 cups grated cabbage
2 carrots, grated
2 stalks celery, sliced
3 cups frozen or canned corn, drained

DRESSING

2 tablespoons corn or safflower oil
4 tablespoons vegetable or chicken broth
½ teaspoon salt
2 teaspoons dijon mustard
2 tablespoons white wine vinegar
½ teaspoon celery seeds
2 scallions, sliced

Mix dressing ingredients together and toss thoroughly, but gently, with the cabbage, carrots, celery, and corn. Chill for a few hours to allow flavors to develop before serving.

Serves 12

NUTRITIVE VALUES PER SERVING:

FAT	FIBER	VIT. A	VIT. C	CAL	CAL FROM FAT
2.67gm	5.35gm	1677 IU	23.3mg	70.1	34%

DILLED CARROTS

*An interesting variation would be to serve these carrots hot, as
a vegetable.*

1½ pounds carrots, sliced

DRESSING

1 tablespoon olive oil

2 tablespoons white wine vinegar

3 tablespoons vegetable or chicken broth

2 teaspoons sugar

½ teaspoon salt

¼ teaspoon pepper

1 teaspoon dried dill weed

¼ cup chopped parsley

Steam carrots until fork-tender. Drain. Combine dressing ingredients, and toss with carrots while they are still warm. (Save
liquid from steaming carrots for soup.)

Marinate carrots for several hours in refrigerator. Serve
chilled.

Serves 6

NUTRITIVE VALUES PER SERVING:

FAT	FIBER	VIT. A	VIT. C	CAL	CAL FROM FAT
2.51gm	5.89gm	12,687 IU	13.7mg	67.1	34%

FRENCH POTATO SALAD

SALAD

8 medium new potatoes (red preferred)
2 carrots, grated
¾ cup chopped green bell pepper
¾ cup chopped red onion

DRESSING

3 tablespoons olive oil
5 tablespoons vegetable or chicken broth
2 tablespoons white wine vinegar
1 tablespoon fresh lemon juice
1½ teaspoons dijon mustard
½ teaspoon salt
¼ teaspoon pepper

Quarter potatoes and steam for 10–15 minutes, depending upon size, until just tender. Cool a bit and cut into bite-sized pieces.

Mix dressing ingredients together and toss in a large bowl with potatoes, carrots, green bell pepper, and onion. Serve chilled or at room temperature.

Serves 10

NUTRITIVE VALUES PER SERVING:

FAT	FIBER	VIT. A	VIT. C	CAL	CAL FROM FAT
4.30gm	4.58gm	1666 IU	42.3mg	165	24%

ICED SUMMER FRUIT SALAD

This is also good as a light dessert.

FRUIT

1 medium cantaloupe, cut into bite-sized pieces
½ medium honeydew melon, cut into bite-sized
  pieces
1 papaya, cut into bite-sized pieces
1 pound seedless grapes

DRESSING

½ cup low-fat yogurt
2 tablespoons apricot preserves
2 tablespoons orange juice

Mix dressing ingredients together and carefully toss with the
fruit. Serve chilled.

Or, for an even more attractive dish, cut melons and papaya
into slices and arrange overlapping on a platter. Sprinkle with
grapes. Drizzle some of the dressing over the fruit and pass the
rest.

Serves 8

NUTRITIVE VALUES PER SERVING:

FAT	FIBER	VIT. A	VIT. C	CAL	CAL FROM FAT
.82gm	2.70gm	2297 IU	55.4mg	111	7%

LEMON-BROCCOLI SALAD

2 pounds broccoli

DRESSING

3 tablespoons vegetable or chicken broth
1½ tablespoons olive oil
3 tablespoons fresh lemon juice
½ teaspoon salt
¼ teaspoon pepper

Separate broccoli into florets. Peel broccoli stems with a paring knife and slice crosswise. Steam broccoli and sliced stems for about 5 minutes, just until fork-tender. Save steaming liquid for soup. Quickly immerse in cold water to stop cooking process. Drain.

Make the dressing by mixing dressing ingredients in a blender. Toss drained broccoli florets and stems with the dressing and marinate for a few hours. Serve chilled.

Serves 6

NUTRITIVE VALUES PER SERVING:

FAT	FIBER	VIT. A	VIT. C	CAL	CAL FROM FAT
1.61gm	9.20gm	3787 IU	141mg	45.6	32%

LENTIL SALAD WITH FETA CHEESE
SALAD

1 cup lentils

3 cups water

1 cup chopped watercress sprigs

2 ounces feta cheese, finely crumbled

DRESSING

2 tablespoons vegetable or chicken broth, fat
  removed

1 tablespoon olive oil

2 tablespoons red wine vinegar

1 clove garlic, minced

¼ teaspoon pepper

½ teaspoon oregano

¼ teaspoon salt

Place lentils in a saucepan; cover with 3 cups of water and bring
to a boil. Simmer for 45 minutes to 1 hour, just until tender
(don't overcook—lentils should not be mushy). Drain well and
cool.

Mix dressing ingredients together in a blender and toss gently
with lentils. Add feta cheese and watercress and lightly toss to
combine well. Serve chilled.

Serves 6

NUTRITIVE VALUES PER SERVING:

FAT	FIBER	VIT. A	VIT. C	CAL	CAL FROM FAT
4.67gm	3.84	260 IU	4.28mg	148	28%

MARINATED BLACK BEAN SALAD

SALAD

1 pound black beans
3 cups cooked brown rice
1 cup chopped onion
1 cup chopped green bell pepper

DRESSING

3 tablespoons corn or safflower oil
3 tablespoons red wine vinegar
3 tablespoons vegetable or chicken broth
1 teaspoon salt
2 teaspoons thyme
½ teaspoon pepper
2 cloves garlic, minced
¼–½ cup chopped fresh cilantro (coriander),
   according to taste (parsley may be
   substituted)

Soak beans overnight and cook according to package directions. Drain well. Mix dressing ingredients together and toss gently with beans, rice, onions, and green bell pepper. Marinate for a few hours to allow flavors to develop. Serve chilled.

Serves 12

NUTRITIVE VALUES PER SERVING:

FAT	FIBER	VIT. A	VIT. C	CAL	CAL FROM FAT
4.14gm	8.18gm	277 IU	21.7mg	153	24%

MEXICAN CHICKEN SALAD

SALAD

1 medium head lettuce (about 12 ounces),
    washed and dried
2 scallions, chopped
1 15-ounce can kidney beans, drained
½ cup chopped green bell pepper
1 cup cooked chicken, chopped

DRESSING

3 tablespoons chicken broth
2 tablespoons corn or safflower oil
2 tablespoons red wine vinegar
1 tablespoon fresh lime juice
1 clove garlic, minced
1½ teaspoons sugar
¾ teaspoon chili powder
½ teaspoon salt
⅓ cup chopped fresh cilantro (coriander)

Shred lettuce and place in a salad bowl. Add scallions, beans, bell
pepper, and chicken.

Make a dressing by mixing dressing ingredients together in a
blender. Just before serving, lightly toss dressing with chicken
salad ingredients. Serve immediately.

Serves 8

NUTRITIVE VALUES PER SERVING:

FAT	FIBER	VIT. A	VIT. C	CAL	CAL FROM FAT
4.50gm	6.44gm	247 IU	16.4mg	138	29%

MOLDED GAZPACHO SALAD

3 cups tomato juice
2 envelopes unflavored gelatin
1 tablespoon sugar
3 tablespoons fresh lemon juice
1½ teaspoons red wine vinegar
¼ teaspoon salt
¼ teaspoon pepper
⅓ cup diced onion
¾ cup diced unpeeled cucumber
½ cup diced celery
¾ cup diced green bell pepper
Lettuce leaves for garnish

Heat tomato juice and stir in gelatin. Heat over medium until gelatin is completely dissolved. Off the heat, add sugar, lemon juice, red wine vinegar, salt, and pepper. Pour into a bowl and chill until thick and syrupy, about 2 hours.

When gelatin is thickened, fold diced vegetables into gelatin mixture and pour into a 6-cup ring mold (or individual cups), coated with cooking spray. Chill until set. Unmold onto lettuce by placing mold briefly into a bowl of warm water and inverting it onto the lettuce-lined plate.

Serves 6

NUTRITIVE VALUES PER SERVING:

FAT	FIBER	VIT. A	VIT. C	CAL	CAL FROM FAT
.20gm	1.60gm	1078 IU	51.0mg	49.9	4%

ORIENTAL TURKEY SALAD
WITH CILANTRO

*With all the ingredients finely chopped, this would make an
excellent filling for sandwiches or a spread for crackers.*

SALAD

2 cups cooked turkey, cut in small cubes (about
   10 ounces)
¾ cup sliced scallions
¾ cup sliced water chestnuts
½ cup sliced celery
½ cup chopped green bell pepper
½ cup chopped parsley
⅓ cup chopped fresh cilantro (coriander)

DRESSING

3 tablespoons chicken broth, fat removed
1 tablespoon mayonnaise
2 tablespoons low-fat yogurt
1 teaspoon Chinese sesame oil
1 teaspoon soy sauce

Combine dressing ingredients and mix with turkey and vegetables. If serving as a salad, an attractive presentation would be to
place a mound of the mixture in a butter lettuce cup.

Serves 6

NUTRITIVE VALUES PER SERVING:

FAT	FIBER	VIT. A	VIT. C	CAL	CAL FROM FAT
4.27gm	2.23gm	762 IU	29.7mg	114	34%

PAPAYA AND CUCUMBER SALAD

SALAD

2 medium papayas, peeled and sliced into bite-sized pieces (save 2 teaspoons papaya seeds for dressing)

1 medium cucumber, sliced (peeling is optional)

6 cups romaine lettuce, washed, dried, and torn into bite-sized pieces

DRESSING

1 tablespoon corn or safflower oil

3 tablespoons white wine vinegar

1 tablespoon sugar

3 tablespoons orange juice

⅛ teaspoon salt

¼ teaspoon dijon mustard

½ teaspoon minced onion

2 teaspoons papaya seeds

Place all dressing ingredients in a blender and process well (until papaya seeds look like specks of pepper). Toss papaya, cucumber, and lettuce in a salad bowl with the dressing and serve immediately.

Serves 8

NUTRITIVE VALUES PER SERVING:

FAT	FIBER	VIT. A	VIT. C	CAL	CAL FROM FAT
1.95gm	1.41gm	1884 IU	42.8mg	53.1	33%

PASTA AND BROCCOLI SALAD

SALAD

¹/₂ pound small whole-wheat pasta shells (white
may be substituted)

1 bunch (about 1 pound) broccoli

1 cup sliced scallions

1 cup chopped green bell pepper

1 cup sliced celery

DRESSING

2 tablespoons corn or safflower oil

5 tablespoons vegetable or chicken broth, fat
removed

5 tablespoons rice wine vinegar or white wine
vinegar

2 tablespoons soy sauce

¹/₂ teaspoon dry mustard

1 teaspoon Chinese sesame oil (found in
Oriental section of market)

Cook pasta according to package directions. Run under cold
water and drain very well.

Break broccoli into florets. Peel stems with paring knife and
slice crosswise. Pour hot water over broccoli florets and stems.
Let stand 5 minutes, then drain well, saving liquid for soup.

Mix dressing ingredients together in a blender. Toss pasta with
dressing. Add broccoli, scallions, green pepper, and celery and
toss to combine. Refrigerate for a few hours and serve chilled.

Serves 10

NUTRITIVE VALUES PER SERVING:

FAT	FIBER	VIT. A	VIT. C	CAL	CAL FROM FAT
3.80gm	6.55gm	1228 IU	63.9mg	141	24%

PASTA SALAD
WITH FRESH TOMATOES

Add leftover chicken or meat, cut in cubes, to make a one-dish meal.

½ **pound small whole-wheat pasta shells (white may be substituted)**

3 **tablespoons olive oil**

2 **cups fresh tomatoes, peeled, seeded, and chopped (to peel and seed, see page 224)**

½ **teaspoon basil**

½ **teaspoon oregano**

2 **cloves garlic, minced**

2 **tablespoons fresh lemon juice**

½ **teaspoon salt**

½ **teaspoon pepper**

1 **cup chopped parsley**

½ **cup chopped red onion**

2 **tablespoons drained capers**

Boil pasta according to package directions. Drain very well and toss with olive oil when dry. Add remaining ingredients and toss gently but thoroughly. Refrigerate for several hours or overnight before serving.

Serves 8

NUTRITIVE VALUES PER SERVING:

FAT	FIBER	VIT. A	VIT. C	CAL	CAL FROM FAT
5.66gm	4.82gm	1059 IU	26.1mg	175	29%

RICE SALAD

With the addition of some cooked seafood or poultry, this could be served as a light entrée.

> **3 cups cooked brown rice (about 1 cup uncooked)**
> **½ teaspoon salt**
> **¼ teaspoon pepper**
> **2 tablespoons mayonnaise**
> **3 tablespoons vegetable or chicken broth**
> **1 teaspoon dijon mustard**
> **⅓ cup sliced scallions**
> **½ cup chopped green bell pepper**
> **2 hard-cooked eggs, chopped**
> **1 tablespoon drained capers**

Cook rice and let it cool. Combine rice with salt, pepper, mayonnaise, broth, and mustard. Toss lightly but thoroughly, mixing all ingredients together. Add other ingredients and gently toss to combine well.

Serve chilled.

Serves 8

Nutritive Values per Serving:

FAT	FIBER	VIT. A	VIT. C	CAL	CAL FROM FAT
4.67gm	1.94gm	113 IU	13.1mg	135	31%

RICE-STUFFED TOMATOES

8 medium-sized tomatoes

3 cups cooked brown rice (about 1 cup uncooked)

⅓ cup chopped scallions

2 tablespoons olive oil

3 tablespoons vegetable or chicken broth

2 tablespoons fresh lemon juice

½ teaspoon oregano

¼ teaspoon salt

¼ teaspoon pepper

Gently press tomatoes on counter so they will stand upright. Carefully remove core with a paring knife. Cut top third off tomatoes and scoop out center, leaving shell intact. Turn upside down to drain, saving pulp.

Chop scooped-out pulp and drain well in a mesh sieve until all the juice is gone (save juice for soup). Finely chop tops of tomatoes. Mix chopped, drained pulp with chopped tops, rice, scallions, oil, broth, lemon juice, oregano, salt, and pepper. Spoon into tomato shells.

Place tomatoes in a small pan with about ⅓ cup water in the bottom. Bake for 15 minutes at 350°F. Cool. May be served chilled or at room temperature.

Serves 8

NUTRITIVE VALUES PER SERVING:

FAT	FIBER	VIT. A	VIT. C	CAL	CAL FROM FAT
4.20gm	3.85gm	1111 IU	30.8mg	146	26%

SALADE NIÇOISE

SALAD

1 large head romaine lettuce
3 medium new potatoes (red preferred)
2 7-ounce cans tuna in water (preferably
   albacore)
½ pound fresh greens beans
3 medium tomatoes, quartered
1 hard-cooked egg, chopped
1 tablespoon drained capers
12 radishes, washed and sliced
½ cup parsley sprigs

DRESSING

3 tablespoons olive oil
5 tablespoons vegetable or chicken broth
4 tablespoons red wine vinegar
1½ scallions, sliced
1½ teaspoons dijon mustard
½ teaspoon salt
¼ teaspoon pepper

Wash lettuce and refrigerate to crisp. Steam potatoes until done, and cut into bite-sized pieces. Drain tuna. Steam green beans until crisp-tender and cut into bite-sized pieces.

Mix dressing ingredients together. Marinate potatoes and beans, separately, each in half of the dressing, for at least 1 hour. Drain, saving dressing.

Line a serving platter with romaine lettuce. Place a mound of potatoes in the center. Place a circle of beans around the potatoes. Place tuna in a circle around the beans. Place tomato quarters, chopped egg, capers, radishes, and parsley sprigs around the other ingredients according to your visual taste and the shape of your platter.

Drizzle reserved dressing over the patter of Salade Niçoise and serve immediately.

Serves 10

NUTRITIVE VALUES PER SERVING:

FAT	FIBER	VIT. A	VIT. C	CAL	CAL FROM FAT
5.49gm	3.28gm	1113 IU	28.5mg	187	26%

SHREDDED CHICKEN SALAD

SALAD

8 ounces cooked chicken breast, torn or cut into shreds

2 tablespoons soy sauce

2 tablespoons sherry

2 scallions, shredded

1 pound Chinese (curly) cabbage, shredded

2 cups cooked brown rice

1 ounce cashews, chopped

¼ cup chopped fresh cilantro (coriander)

1 8-ounce can water chestnuts, drained and sliced

DRESSING

½ cup chicken broth

2 teaspoons corn or safflower oil

2 teaspoons Chinese sesame oil (from Oriental section of market)

¼ teaspoon dry mustard

Marinate chicken in soy sauce and sherry for ½ hour. Shred scallions by cutting across into thirds, then slicing lengthwise.

Make the dressing by combining dressing ingredients in a blender. Just before serving, toss the chicken and its marinade, scallions, cabbage, rice, cashews, cilantro, and water chestnuts with the dressing. Serve immediately.

Serves 8 as a salad

NUTRITIVE VALUES PER SERVING:

FAT	FIBER	VIT. A	VIT. C	CAL	CAL FROM FAT
3.76gm	3.96gm	1764 IU	16.0mg	107	32%

SPINACH AND GRAPEFRUIT SALAD

SALAD

2 large bunches fresh spinach, washed and
dried, stems removed

3 medium red grapefruits, peeled and cut into
bite-sized pieces

DRESSING

1 tablespoon toasted sesame seeds

2 tablespoons vegetable or chicken broth

1 tablespoon corn or safflower oil

1 tablespoon white wine vinegar

1 tablespoon fresh lemon juice

1 tablespoon honey

¼ teaspoon pepper

¼ teaspoon salt

To toast sesame seeds, heat for 5 minutes in an ungreased frying
pan on medium heat, tossing frequently, until golden brown.

Mix dressing ingredients together in a blender. Just before
serving, toss spinach and grapefruit with the dressing.

Serves 8

NUTRITIVE VALUES PER SERVING:

FAT	FIBER	VIT. A	VIT. C	CAL	CAL FROM FAT
2.63gm	7.07gm	6929 IU	77.9mg	79.6	30%

SPINACH SALAD SUPREME

SALAD

1 large or 2 medium bunches fresh spinach
2 medium red potatoes, steamed until done, chopped
1 hard-cooked egg, chopped
2 tablespoons sunflower seeds
1 scallion, sliced
2 carrots, grated

DRESSING

½ cup low-fat yogurt
1 tablespoon red wine vinegar
¼ teaspoon tarragon
½ teaspoon salt
¼ teaspoon pepper
½ teaspoon sugar
¼ teaspoon basil
1 tablespoon finely chopped scallions

Wash and dry spinach and place in refrigerator to crisp.

Mix dressing ingredients together in a blender. Just before serving, toss all the salad ingredients with the dressing.

Or, for an especially attractive dish, place spinach on a plate and garnish with potatoes, egg, sunflower seeds, scallions, and carrots arranged in a circular pattern over the spinach. Drizzle dressing over Spinach Salad Platter. Serve immediately.

Serves 6

NUTRITIVE VALUES PER SERVING:

FAT	FIBER	VIT. A	VIT. C	CAL	CAL FROM FAT
2.94gm	6.83gm	7207 IU	41.6mg	117	23%

SUMMER SALAD

SALAD

2 cups frozen or canned corn, drained

½ pound ripe tomatoes, cored and cut into
  eighths, lengthwise

½ pound zucchini, sliced

⅔ cup sliced scallions

½ pound green bell pepper, quartered and sliced

DRESSING

¼ cup buttermilk

1 tablespoon low-fat yogurt

1 tablespoon mayonnaise

2 tablespoons vegetable or chicken broth

1 clove garlic, minced

½ teaspoon dijon mustard

¼ teaspoon paprika

¼ teaspoon salt

¼ teaspoon oregano

2 tablespoons finely chopped parsley

Mix dressing ingredients together. Gently toss vegetables with dressing, being careful not to break or crush vegetables. Serve chilled.

Serves 6

NUTRITIVE VALUES PER SERVING:

FAT	FIBER	VIT. A	VIT. C	CAL	CAL FROM FAT
2.55gm	5.59gm	827 IU	70.4mg	93.2	25%

TACO SALAD

This salad has such a variety of flavor and texture, and is so moist, that we find it to be delicious without a dressing. We have suggested a dressing for those who want it, but the salad will be higher in fat.

1 pound lean ground round
3 cups kidney beans, drained
1 teaspoon chili powder
¾ cup Tangy French Dressing (see Index)(optional)*
1 large head romaine lettuce
4 scallions, sliced
6 tomatoes, chopped
3 ounces part-skim mozzarella cheese, grated
1½ cups chopped green bell pepper
1 cup Tortilla Chips, broken (see Index)

Without any fat in the pan, cook ground round until crumbly and cooked through. Drain very well. Add kidney beans and chili powder; cook 5 minutes more. Just before serving, add Tangy French Dressing and heat through.

Place lettuce, scallions, tomatoes, cheese, and bell pepper in a large salad bowl. When ready to serve, toss with beef-bean mixture and sprinkle with Tortilla Chips. Serve immediately.

Serves 12

*NUTRITIVE VALUES PER SERVING (determined without the dressing):

FAT	FIBER	VIT. A	VIT. C	CAL	CAL FROM FAT
5.11gm	6.60gm	1291 IU	44.3mg	164	28%

TANGY CARROT SALAD

3 large carrots, grated

2 cups cooked brown rice

3 scallions, sliced

1 teaspoon fresh minced ginger*

2 tablespoons corn or safflower oil

2 tablespoons fresh lemon juice

2 tablespoons vegetable or chicken broth

½ teaspoon salt

½ teaspoon sugar

Combine carrots, rice, scallions, and ginger in a salad bowl. Make a dressing by combining oil, lemon juice, broth, salt, and sugar. Toss dressing with vegetables and marinate a few hours. Serve chilled.

Serves 6

---

*There is no good substitute for fresh ginger. If it is unavailable, add an extra half scallion, chopped, and ¼ teaspoon cayenne pepper.

NUTRITIVE VALUES PER SERVING:

FAT	FIBER	VIT. A	VIT. C	CAL	CAL FROM FAT
5.19gm	4.34gm	5380 IU	9.74mg	144	33%

TOMATO AND WATERCRESS SALAD

SALAD

2 cups watercress, washed, stems removed

3 medium red potatoes, steamed until done, sliced

3 large fresh tomatoes, sliced

¾ cup coarsely chopped fresh basil, stems removed

1 medium red onion, thinly sliced, separated into rings

DRESSING

2 tablespoons olive oil

3 tablespoons vegetable or chicken broth

2 tablespoons fresh lemon juice

1 tablespoon red wine vinegar

2 teaspoons dijon mustard

1 clove garlic, minced

Arrange watercress on a serving plate. Alternate sliced potatoes with tomato slices on top of the watercress. Sprinkle with fresh basil and decorate with onion slices. (This salad may also be arranged on 6 individual dishes.)

Combine dressing ingredients in a blender. Drizzle dressing over the arranged vegetables. Serve immediately.

Serves 6

NUTRITIVE VALUES PER SERVING:

FAT	FIBER	VIT. A	VIT. C	CAL	CAL FROM FAT
4.76gm	3.66gm	830 IU	37.9mg	134	32%

VEGETABLE SALAD

SALAD

1 medium head broccoli

1 medium cucumber, peeled, grated, and
   drained

2 carrots, grated

DRESSING

¾ cup low-fat yogurt

½ teaspoon dill

¼ teaspoon salt

¼ cup chopped scallions

¼ cup chopped green bell pepper

1 tablespoon fresh lemon juice

Break broccoli into very small florets; peel and thinly slice stems with a paring knife. Cover broccoli florets and stems with boiling water and let sit for 5 minutes. Drain broccoli well. (Reserve liquid for soup or other uses.)

Combine broccoli, cucumbers, and carrots in a salad bowl. Mix dressing ingredients together and gently toss with the vegetables. Serve chilled or at room temperature.

Serves 6

NUTRITIVE VALUES PER SERVING:

FAT	FIBER	VIT. A	VIT. C	CAL	CAL FROM FAT
.75gm	5.94gm	4627 IU	80.9mg	46.5	15%

WHITE BEAN SALAD

SALAD

1 pound white beans
1 cup chopped red onion
½ cup chopped parsley

DRESSING

3 tablespoons olive oil
6 tablespoons broth
3 tablespoons red wine vinegar
2 cloves garlic, minced
2 teaspoons oregano
½ teaspoon salt
½ teaspoon pepper

Cook beans according to package directions; drain gently but well.

Mix dressing ingredients together and gently toss with beans, onions, and parsley. Marinate for several hours. Serve chilled.

Serves 10

NUTRITIVE VALUES PER SERVING:

FAT	FIBER	VIT. A	VIT. C	CAL	CAL FROM FAT
5.29gm	2.44gm	262 IU	6.85mg	202	24%

4
Seafood, Poultry, and Meat

SEAFOOD

Adriatic Fish Fillets
Clams Steamed in Wine
Fillet of Sole Braised in Lettuce
Fish Dijon
Flounder Creole
Linguini with Clam Sauce
Lobster Tails Italiano
Mediterranean Fish Stew
Teriyaki Halibut

POULTRY

Chicken and Sweet Potatoes
Chicken Bouillabaisse
Chicken Breasts in Foil
Chicken Fettucine
Chicken Scaloppine
Chicken-Spinach Salad Platter
Chicken with Grapes and Mushrooms
Crispy Parmesan Chicken
Curried Turkey and Broccoli
Jambalaya
Mandarin Orange Chicken with Broccoli
Mustard Sauce Turkey with
  Brussels Sprouts
Perfectly Poached Chicken
Spicy Sesame Noodles with Turkey
  and Scallops

Sweet and Sour Chicken with Vegetables
Turkey Breast with Lemon and
  Cauliflower
Turkey Chili with Garnishes

MEAT

Corned Beef (without nitrates)
Country Sausage and Potatoes
Creole Sausage with Rice and Beans
French Beef with Vegetables
French Veal Ragout
Greek Meatballs
Italian Sausages
Mexican-Style Beef Stew
Oven-Roasted Lamb with
  Vegetable Sauce
Portuguese Cabbage Rolls
Ragout of Lamb
Sausage and Peppers Italiano
South American Chili Beef in Tortillas
Southern Beef Loaf
Spinach-Stuffed Flank Steak
Stuffed Peppers California
Veal Chorizo
Veal-Rice Stroganoff
Veal Roast Royale
Veal Stroganoff Madeira
Venetian Liver

Seafood, Poultry, and Meat

When it's time to prepare the main course, there are many types of seafood, poultry, and meat to choose from on a cancer risk–reduction eating plan. The focus in this chapter is to keep fat to a minimum, and flavor and creativity to a maximum. Working with such favorites as lobster; chicken breasts; scallops; white meat of turkey; lean sirloin and other lean cuts of beef, veal, and lamb; and some wonderfully light fish, these recipes are tasty and inviting, and will appeal to a wide variety of appetites.

The entrées are designed so that one entrée serving is approximately 3 ounces of meat, or 4 ounces of seafood or poultry. (This supplies the average adult female about 62% of her daily protein requirement, and the adult male about 49%.) *Be sure to adhere to this portion size*, because lean meats, seafood, and poultry *still* contain 9–35% calories from fat.

Use the following guidelines to plan your menus:

- Eat most often: white meat of turkey (with skin removed); white fish (halibut, flounder, sole, perch, shark, swordfish); water-packed tuna or salmon; chicken breasts (with fat pockets and skin removed); shellfish such as clams or mussels; lobster, veal, and scaloppine.

- Eat in moderation: lean sirloin of beef, ground round steak, dark meat of chicken and turkey, pink or red salmon (fresh or frozen), flank steak, lean cuts of lamb, lean cuts of veal (steaks and chops).
- Eat only occasionally: beef roasts, lean pork, veal roasts, lamb chops.

It is worth the time to find a good butcher who will help you select the best lean cuts of meat and then also trim the visible fat. The latter service alone will save you a good amount of preparation time. Then use the cooking methods described below to ensure tenderness.

COOKING METHODS

One basic cooking rule for all meat, seafood, and poultry: never overcook. Besides giving a tough, hard texture, overcooking ruins the taste.

Fish

The most popular methods of cooking fish are *broiling* or *sautéing* because of the delicate texture of fish. Both methods take only a few minutes on each side until the fish becomes opaque. Sauté in a scant amount of oil or margarine, or better, use a nonfat cooking spray in a treated pan. To *poach* firm-fleshed fish, put into simmering liquid (wine, juices, or broth) for about 8–10 minutes, or until fish becomes opaque. You can *bake* fish wrapped in foil, wrapped in lettuce leaves (see Fillet of Sole Braised in Lettuce), or placed in a lightly oiled dish with a small amount of liquid. These methods of baking all ensure that the fish will not dry out. To bake any fish, preheat the oven to 400–450°F. Allow 10 minutes cooking time per inch of thickness of fish. If you are going to stuff the fish, measure the thickness after it has been stuffed. To avoid that occasional "fishy" smell in the house, soak fresh or frozen fish fillets in milk overnight in the refrigerator.

Chicken

Whole chicken may be *roasted* at 350°F for 18–20 minutes per pound. Baste often and remove skin before serving. You may also *poach* chicken pieces using the recipe for Perfectly Poached Chicken in this chapter.

Small chickens or game hens may be cut in half and *broiled* for 15 minutes on each side. Baste with broth 2 or 3 times. Or thinly slice chicken breasts into scaloppine and *sauté* (see Chicken Scaloppine, this chapter).

Chicken may also be *braised.* Braising is a combination of browning, stewing, and steaming, rendering a tender, moist dish. Lightly brown one cut up chicken in a small amount of margarine, add some broth, cover, and cook slowly on stove top or in the oven at 325°F for 1½ to 2 hours.

Turkey

The most popular and easiest way to cook turkey is to *roast* it whole. Place bird breast-side up in a large roasting pan and put into an oven preheated to 325°F. Cooking on low heat keeps it from drying out. Baste often with pan juices. An 8–12 pound bird should cook for 3½ to 4 hours; turkey is done when you pierce the thigh and the juices run clear. Remember to remove the skin before serving.

Turkey may also be cut into pieces and *poached.* Follow the procedure in our recipe for Perfectly Poached Chicken, except use a bigger pot. This is a good way to cook turkey for a party.

Use the breast meat for sandwiches or roll warm slices around asparagus or broccoli spears. Cover with one of our light sauces such as Thyme Sauce. Use the dark meat of the turkey for kabobs, add to stir-fried dishes, or combine with white meat for turkey salad.

Beef

Beef may be *braised* using the method described for braising chicken. This is particularly good for lean cuts of beef such as top round. It can also be cut into thin strips and used in stir-fried dishes, or you can stuff and *bake* it as in our Spinach-Stuffed Flank Steak.

Sirloin tip may be *broiled,* cut into pieces for kabobs, or thinly sliced for stroganoff. (See Veal Stroganoff Madeira; you can substitute very lean beef strips for veal.)

Stew meat can be cut from any lean part of the beef. Cover and cook slowly in liquid to prevent it from becoming too tough.

Enhance plain meat, fish, or poultry with sauces from Chapter

8. Try Creamy Caper-Mustard Sauce or Ginger Sauce for poultry; Lemon Yogurt Sauce or Thyme Sauce on fish; Horseradish Cream or Spanish Vegetable Sauce with beef; Mint Sauce or Dill Sauce on lean lamb; and Mushroom Sauce and Madeira Sauce on veal slices.

Many of our entrées are complete meals in themselves: French Beef with Vegetables, Turkey Breast with Lemon and Cauliflower, Jambalaya, and Sweet and Sour Chicken with Vegetables.

If you can't live without fried chicken, try Crispy Parmesan Chicken. Remove the skin, brush with a small amount of oil and dijon mustard, coat with a mixture of bread crumbs and parmesan cheese, and bake to a crispy perfection (without the enormous amount of fat that goes with regular fried chicken).

Southern Beef Loaf turns a ho-hum dish into a light and delicious entrée using a bit of applesauce as the secret flavor ingredient. Leftovers are great for sandwiches and they don't have those surprise fat deposits you usually encounter in cold meat loaf.

Fillet of Sole Braised in Lettuce, Oven-Roasted Lamb with Vegetables, Lobster Tails Italiano, and Spinach-Stuffed Flank Steak are among the entrées that would be considered "company fare," as would ethnic dishes such as Greek Meatballs, Sausage and Peppers Italiano, Mediterranean Fish Stew, and Veal Stroganoff Madeira.

Chili fans will love Turkey Chili with Garnishes. It has an authentic Tex-Mex flavor, but compared to regular commercial chili has 50% less fat. And for the busy cook, some fast and simple entrées include Fish Dijon, Chicken Breasts in Foil, and French Veal Ragout, all taking less than thirty minutes to prepare from the time you enter the kitchen.

As you can see, the recipes in this chapter are varied, interesting, and most important, low in fat. And because the choices are so plentiful and flavorful, you will find the switch from high-fat to lower-fat dishes a pleasure.

ADRIATIC FISH FILLETS

1 tablespoon margarine or butter, melted
1 tablespoon olive oil
2 tablespoons fresh lemon juice
1 tablespoon vegetable or chicken broth
½ teaspoon thyme
½ teaspoon basil
¼ cup chopped fresh parsley
1 clove garlic, minced
½ teaspoon salt
¼ teaspoon pepper
1 pound fish fillets

Melt margarine and combine with oil, lemon juice, broth, thyme, basil, parsley, garlic, salt, and pepper in a 9″ × 13″ baking dish. Place fish in oil mixture in a single layer; turn to coat. Let stand 30 minutes.

Preheat oven to 350°F. Turn fish again, then bake, covered, for 15 minutes at 350°F. Lift fish out of liquid in pan and serve immediately.

Serves 4

NUTRITIVE VALUES PER SERVING:

FAT	FIBER	VIT. A	VIT. C	CAL	CAL FROM FAT
4.75gm	.36gm	380 IU	8.19mg	135	32%

CLAMS STEAMED IN WINE

9 pounds clams
1 cup cornmeal
3 tablespoons margarine or butter
1½ cups finely chopped onion
3 cloves garlic, minced
¾ cup chopped fresh parsley
3 cups dry white wine
⅓ cup freshly grated parmesan cheese

Scrub clams well to remove surface dirt. Place clams in a bowl of cold water to which cornmeal has been added. Swish clams around and soak for 30 minutes. Remove clams from water.

Melt margarine in a large kettle; stir in onion and garlic and cook slowly for 4 or 5 minutes, until wilted. Add parsley and clams. Cover kettle and shake gently to mix clams and other ingredients. Pour in wine and shake gently again. Turn heat to high, cover tightly, reduce heat, and steam until all the clams are open (about 5 minutes). Clams are done as soon as they open.

Transfer clams to a large serving bowl or individual bowls. Divide the liquid among servings and sprinkle with parmesan. Serve with crusty whole grain bread or Garlic Herb Bread (see Index) to dip in the wonderful broth!

Serves 6

NUTRITIVE VALUES PER SERVING:

FAT	FIBER	VIT. A	VIT. C	CAL	CAL FROM FAT
9.03gm	1.36gm	927 IU	20.5mg	270	30%

FILLET OF SOLE
BRAISED IN LETTUCE

6 large butter lettuce leaves
6 4-ounce boneless fillets of sole
½ teaspoon salt
¼ teaspoon pepper
1½ tablespoons margarine or butter
6 tablespoons sliced scallions
1 teaspoon corn or safflower oil

Blanch lettuce in simmering water for 40 seconds. Place in cold water, gently drain, and dry, trying to keep leaves whole. Sprinkle each fillet with salt and pepper. Dot with margarine and scallions. Wrap each fillet in a blanched lettuce leaf. Place seam side down on a lightly oiled pan. Brush each lettuce-wrapped fillet lightly with oil to prevent drying.

Bake about 7 minutes in a preheated 375°F oven. Serve with Thyme Sauce (see Index).

Serves 6

Nutritive Values per Serving:

FAT	FIBER	VIT. A	VIT. C	CAL	CAL FROM FAT
4.7gm	.4gm	379 IU	3.86mg	146	30%

FISH DIJON

1 pound boneless fish fillets
2 teaspoons dijon mustard
⅓ cup chopped fresh parsley
⅓ cup chopped red onion
⅓ cup chopped green bell pepper
½ cup cooked brown rice
⅓ cup fish or chicken stock
½ cup grated part-skim mozzarella cheese
⅓ cup bread crumbs
Paprika

Place half the fish in a single layer in an 8″ × 8″ pan coated with cooking spray. Spread fish with mustard. Sprinkle fish with parsley, onion, green pepper, and rice. Place remaining fish fillets over the rice filling. Pour stock over fish and sprinkle with cheese. Cover with bread crumbs and sprinkle with paprika.

Bake, covered, in a preheated 350°F oven for 15 minutes. Serve immediately.

Serves 4

NUTRITIVE VALUES PER SERVING:

FAT	FIBER	VIT. A	VIT. C	CAL	CAL FROM FAT
4.69gm	1.39gm	583 IU	21.6mg	222	19%

FLOUNDER CREOLE

1 cup uncooked brown rice

1 pound fillet of flounder (sole may be substituted)

1 cup chopped onion

1 cup chopped green bell pepper

1 cup chopped tomatoes

¼ cup white wine

½ teaspoon salt

½ teaspoon basil

¼ teaspoon pepper

Start rice, cooking according to package directions, about 15 minutes before preparing fish.

Place fish in a large pan with a cover. Arrange onion, green pepper, and tomatoes around fish. Pour wine over fish. Sprinkle with salt, basil, and pepper. Cover and cook over medium-low heat for 10 minutes, or until fish is opaque and cooked through.

Arrange fish on a platter surrounded by rice. Spoon sauce and vegetables over both fish and rice.

Serves 4

NUTRITIVE VALUES PER SERVING:

FAT	FIBER	VIT. A	VIT. C	CAL	CAL FROM FAT
2.91gm	4.94gm	573 IU	18.2mg	315	8%

LINGUINI WITH CLAM SAUCE

18 ounces linguini, uncooked
3 7½-ounce cans chopped clams
5 teaspoons olive oil
2 tablespoons margarine or butter
1 cup finely chopped carrots
½ cup finely sliced scallions
2 large cloves garlic, minced
1 cup bottled or canned clam juice
1 cup low-fat milk
½ cup finely chopped parsley
¼ teaspoon pepper

Boil linguini according to package directions. While linguini is cooking, prepare clam sauce.

Drain clams and reserve juice. Heat oil and margarine in a large skillet and sauté carrots for 5 minutes. Add scallions and garlic and cook for 5 minutes (don't brown). Add juice from canned clams, 1 cup bottled juice, and milk. Boil for 10 minutes.

Just before serving, add clams, parsley, and pepper to the sauce. Bring sauce to a boil and pour over hot linguini. Serve immediately.

Serves 8

NUTRITIVE VALUES PER SERVING:

FAT	FIBER	VIT. A	VIT. C	CAL	CAL FROM FAT
12.9gm	2.77gm	3666 IU	11.0mg	378	31%

LOBSTER TAILS ITALIANO

8 3- to 4-ounce lobster tails, fresh or frozen
2 tablespoons fresh lemon juice
2 tablespoons margarine or butter
1 tablespoon olive oil
1 cup finely chopped onions
½ cup finely chopped green bell pepper
1 cup chopped fresh tomatoes
2 garlic cloves, minced
¼ cup chopped fresh parsley
½ teaspoon basil
½ teaspoon oregano
¼ teaspoon salt
¼ teaspoon pepper

Drop lobster tails into enough boiling water to cover. Bring to a second boil. Add lemon juice and simmer 3–5 minutes (depending on whether lobsters are fresh or frozen). Lobster meat is done when it turns opaque.

With a scissors or knife, cut away membrane on underside of tail. Pull lobster meat out of shells, starting at the wide part of the tail. Keep shells in one piece for stuffing later. Cut lobster meat into small cubes.

Melt margarine and olive oil in a heavy pan. Sauté onions and green pepper for 3 minutes. Add tomatoes, garlic, parsley, basil, and oregano and simmer, uncovered, for 20 minutes. Add salt, pepper, and lobster cubes. Remove from heat and stir to combine all ingredients. At this point, the lobster mixture may be served hot over rice, or baked in the lobster shells.

To bake in shells, preheat oven to 375°F. Put the shells in baking dish, and divide lobster mixture among them, to overflowing, if necessary. Cook tails at 375°F for 10 minutes or until bubbly. If made ahead and refrigerated, cook for 15 minutes. Serve with 1 slice french or italian bread per person.

Serves 8

Nutritive Values per Serving:

FAT	FIBER	VIT. A	VIT. C	CAL	CAL FROM FAT
7.42gm	1.29gm	607 IU	27.1mg	232	29%

MEDITERRANEAN FISH STEW

With crusty whole grain bread to dip in the broth, and a salad on the side, this makes a wonderful meal!

HERB WINE BROTH

4 teaspoons olive oil

1¼ cups chopped onion

2 cloves garlic, minced

2 medium carrots, finely chopped

1 medium tomato, peeled, seeded, and chopped
  (to peel and seed, see page 224)

½ teaspoon basil

½ teaspoon thyme

3½ cups chicken broth

3 8-ounce bottles clam juice

1 cup dry white wine

1½ teaspoons grated orange peel

STEW

8 clams in the shell

2 pounds assorted fresh firm fish, cut into bite-
  sized chunks (such as halibut or swordfish)

½ cup chopped fresh parsley

4 lemons, cut in half

To make herb wine broth, heat olive oil in a large pan. Sauté onion, garlic, and carrots until onion is limp. Stir in tomato, basil, thyme, broth, clam juice, wine, and orange peel. Cover and simmer 30 minutes. Broth may be used immediately, but is even better if made a day or two ahead and refrigerated until use.

To assemble stew, bring broth to boiling in a large pot. Stir in clams and fish. Bring to a second boil, reduce heat, cover, and simmer over medium heat until clams have opened (about 5–10 minutes). Ladle broth into bowls and divide fish and clams among bowls. Garnish each serving with parsley and lemon wedges.

Serves 8

NUTRITIVE VALUES PER SERVING:

FAT	FIBER	VIT. A	VIT. C	CAL	CAL FROM FAT
6.63gm	2.03gm	2553 IU	21.9mg	206	29%

TERIYAKI HALIBUT

1 pound halibut
¼ cup soy sauce
¼ cup sherry
2 tablespoons Chinese sesame oil (found in
    Oriental section of market)
1 cup raw brown rice

Marinate halibut in soy sauce, sherry, and sesame oil for 12 hours or overnight.

About 45 minutes before cooking halibut, start rice, cooking according to package directions. Bake halibut in marinade sauce at 350°F for 15 minutes, turning every 5 minutes. The baking time depends on the thickness of the fish—don't overcook or the fish will be dry. As soon as the fish has turned opaque it is done. Serve with hot rice, spooning some of the sauce over each portion of rice.

Serves 4

NUTRITIVE VALUES PER SERVING:

FAT	FIBER	VIT. A	VIT. C	CAL	CAL FROM FAT
11.3gm	3.15gm	68.6 IU	0	357	29%

CHICKEN AND SWEET POTATOES

1 pound boneless, skinless chicken breast, cut in 1-inch cubes

2 cups unpeeled sweet potatoes, cut in 1-inch cubes

2 cups carrots, cut in 1-inch cubes

½ cup orange juice

½ cup water

½ teaspoon garlic powder

¼ teaspoon ground ginger

1 teaspoon honey

¼ cup chopped fresh parsley

1 orange, peeled and sliced

Cut chicken, potatoes, and carrots into cubes of approximately the same size and place in a casserole. Combine orange juice, water, garlic powder, ginger, and honey and pour over chicken and vegetables. Cover tightly.

Bake for 1 hour in a preheated 350°F oven. Sprinkle with parsley and garnish with orange slices. Serve immediately.

Serves 6

NUTRITIVE VALUES PER SERVING:

FAT	FIBER	VIT. A	VIT. C	CAL	CAL FROM FAT
2.43gm	4.48gm	8793 IU	36.4mg	185	12%

CHICKEN BOUILLABAISSE

8 halved chicken breasts, boned and skinned
3 tablespoons olive oil
2 cups thinly sliced onions
3 cloves garlic, minced
3 cups chopped fresh tomatoes (or drained
**   canned tomatoes)**
¼ cup tomato sauce
½ teaspoon fennel seeds
1½ teaspoons thyme
3 bay leaves
¼ teaspoon sugar
½ teaspoon salt
¼ teaspoon pepper
1½ cups white wine
½ cup chopped fresh parsley

Sauté chicken in olive oil over medium heat for 10 minutes, turning several times. Remove chicken from pan, leaving oil residue. Add onions and garlic and cook over low heat for 5 minutes (don't brown). Add tomatoes, tomato sauce, fennel, thyme, bay leaves, sugar, salt, and pepper, stirring to combine. Arrange chicken in pan; spoon tomato mixture over chicken. Cook 10 minutes, covered.

Turn chicken pieces over; add wine and bring to a boil. Reduce heat and simmer, covered, 15 minutes more. Remove chicken and keep warm in oven. Boil sauce over medium-high heat for about 10 minutes, until sauce is thickened a bit. Arrange chicken on a platter or on individual plates. Cover with sauce and sprinkle with parsley.

Serves 8

NUTRITIVE VALUES PER SERVING:

FAT	FIBER	VIT. A	VIT. C	CAL	CAL FROM FAT
7.87gm	3.25gm	1329 IU	33.3mg	234	30%

CHICKEN BREASTS IN FOIL

6 halved chicken breasts, boned and skinned
4 cups boiling water
2 cups julienne-cut carrots (matchstick size)
5 teaspoons margarine or butter
2 tablespoons flour
$\frac{1}{2}$ teaspoon salt
$\frac{1}{8}$ teaspoon pepper
$\frac{1}{8}$ teaspoon cayenne pepper
$\frac{1}{4}$ teaspoon nutmeg
$\frac{1}{4}$ cup sliced scallions
$\frac{1}{2}$ cup low-fat milk
$\frac{1}{2}$ cup chicken broth
$\frac{1}{2}$ cup white wine

Poach chicken by placing in a pan of 4 cups of rapidly boiling water. Cover pan and remove from heat. Let chicken set in water for 10 minutes off heat (don't uncover during the 10-minute period).

Steam carrots for about 3 minutes, just until tender. Melt margarine; add flour, salt, pepper, cayenne, and nutmeg, and cook until smooth and golden, stirring constantly. Add scallions and cook for 5 minutes. Add milk and broth; bring to a boil, reduce heat, and simmer 5 minutes. Off heat, blend in wine; return to stove and heat through.

Preheat oven to 350°F. Place a chicken breast on each of 6 10" × 12" pieces of foil. Cover each with $\frac{1}{6}$ of the carrots and sauce. Fold to tightly enclose ingredients. Bake for 20 minutes at 350°F.

Serves 6

NUTRITIVE VALUES PER SERVING:

FAT	FIBER	VIT. A	VIT. C	CAL	CAL FROM FAT
6.32gm	2.47gm	5700 IU	4.54mg	194	29%

CHICKEN FETTUCINE

10 ounces whole-wheat fettuccine (white may
    be substituted)

1 tablespoon margarine or butter

¼ cup white wine

½ pound boneless, skinless chicken breast, cut
    in small pieces

1 cup sliced fresh mushrooms

1 cup grated carrots

1 tablespoon margarine or butter (additional)

2 tablespoons flour

1½ cups low-fat milk

¼ teaspoon oregano

¼ teaspoon thyme

¼ teaspoon basil

½ teaspoon salt

½ teaspoon pepper

½ cup chopped fresh parsley

2 tablespoons freshly grated parmesan cheese

½ cup sliced scallions

Boil fettuccine while preparing chicken and vegetables. When
done, drain fettuccine and keep warm.

Heat 1 tablespoon margarine and the wine in a skillet until
margarine melts. Add chicken, mushrooms, and carrots and
sauté for 5 minutes, or until chicken is cooked. Remove chicken
and vegetables to a bowl and keep warm.

Melt 1 tablespoon (additional) margarine in skillet. Add flour
and cook, stirring, until golden brown. Add milk; bring to a boil,
lower heat, and whisk until blended and thickened. Stir in
oregano, thyme, basil, salt, pepper, and parsley and toss with the
hot, drained fettuccine and the vegetable mixture. Sprinkle with
parmesan and scallions and serve immediately.

Serves 6

NUTRITIVE VALUES PER SERVING:

FAT	FIBER	VIT. A	VIT. C	CAL	CAL FROM FAT
6.95gm	7.54gm	3604 IU	13.7mg	211	30%

CHICKEN SCALOPPINE

This is simple and delicious.

1 pound raw chicken breasts, cut into thin "scaloppine" slices
2 tablespoons margarine or butter
¼ cup dry white wine
2 tablespoons chicken broth
1 tablespoon lemon juice
2 teaspoons capers
2 cups cooked brown rice (about ⅔ cup raw)

Sauté chicken scaloppine slices in margarine, over medium-high heat, for about 1 minute on each side, until barely done. Remove chicken and keep warm. Add the wine, broth, and lemon juice to the pan and boil over medium-high heat for 3 minutes to reduce sauce a bit, scraping bottom of pan to incorporate browned particles into the sauce.

Add the capers and return chicken to pan, turning chicken to coat with sauce. Simmer over low heat for 5 minutes.

Serve chicken alongside the cooked rice (start cooking rice about 20 minutes before beginning chicken recipe, so they will be done at the same time). Spoon some of the sauce over the rice.

Serves 4

NUTRITIVE VALUES PER SERVING:

FAT	FIBER	VIT. A	VIT. C	CAL	CAL FROM FAT
9.36gm	2.25gm	252 IU	0	309	29%

CHICKEN-SPINACH SALAD PLATTER

Quantities may easily be increased to feed more people.

1 bunch fresh spinach, washed and dried

6 ounces boneless, skinless, cooked chicken breast, sliced

1 unpeeled cucumber, thinly sliced

2 carrots, julienne-cut (matchstick size)

2 oranges, peeled and sliced

2 scallions, sliced

8 sprigs fresh cilantro (coriander)

⅓ recipe Creamy Soy Dressing (see Index)

Divide spinach between 2 dinner plates. Arrange slices of chicken down the center. Arrange cucumber, carrots, and oranges attractively on top of spinach. Sprinkle with scallions and sprigs of cilantro.

Drizzle with Creamy Soy Dressing just before serving.

Serves 2

NUTRITIVE VALUES PER SERVING:

FAT	FIBER	VIT. A	VIT. C	CAL	CAL FROM FAT
11.2gm	12.8gm	15,481 IU	128mg	339	30%

CHICKEN WITH
GRAPES AND MUSHROOMS

1 tablespoon unbleached white flour
¼ teaspoon salt
¼ teaspoon pepper
2 pounds boneless, skinless chicken breasts, cut
  into bite-sized pieces
3 tablespoons margarine or butter
¼ cup minced onion
½ pound small fresh mushrooms (or larger ones,
  quartered)
¾ cup chicken broth
½ cup white wine
½ cup low-fat milk
1 tablespoon cornstarch
1 tablespoon water
1 cup seedless grapes

Mix flour, salt, and pepper; coat chicken pieces by shaking in a bag with flour mixture.

Heat margarine in a skillet and sauté chicken until lightly browned. Transfer chicken with a slotted spoon to a casserole dish. Add minced onion to skillet and cook over low heat until onion is softened (add a bit of broth to skillet if margarine has been absorbed by chicken). Add mushrooms and cook over low heat for about 3 minutes. Remove onions and mushrooms with a slotted spoon and add to cooked chicken in casserole.

Add broth and wine to skillet and bring to a boil. Add milk, bring to a second boil, and simmer over medium-high heat for 5 minutes. Mix cornstarch and water and add to the simmering sauce, whisking constantly; remove as soon as sauce is thickened.

Add sauce to chicken and mushrooms and bake in covered casserole for 20 minutes in a preheated 325°F oven. Add grapes and bake another 10 minutes at 325°F. Serve immediately.

Serves 8

NUTRITIVE VALUES PER SERVING:

FAT	FIBER	VIT. A	VIT. C	CAL	CAL FROM FAT
8.02gm	2.16gm	242 IU	3.87mg	232	31%

CRISPY PARMESAN CHICKEN

6 halved chicken breasts, boned and skinned
¾ cup dried bread crumbs
3 tablespoons freshly grated parmesan cheese
1 teaspoon oregano
½ teaspoon salt
⅓ cup chopped parsley
2 tablespoons margarine or butter
2 tablespoons chicken broth, fat removed
2 cloves garlic, minced
1 teaspoon dijon mustard
½ teaspoon worcestershire sauce

Remove any fat from chicken. Combine bread crumbs, parmesan, oregano, salt, and parsley.

Melt margarine with broth: add garlic, mustard, and worcestershire to margarine. Cook on medium heat for 5 minutes. Cool slightly.

Preheat oven to 375°F. Dip chicken into margarine mixture, then roll in bread crumb mixture to coat well, patting bread crumbs firmly onto chicken pieces. Place on a lightly oiled baking tray (don't crowd pieces). Bake for 20 minutes at 375°F, then turn over with a metal spatula (a metal spatula won't dislodge any crumbs from the chicken). Bake another 20 minutes and serve immediately.

Serves 6

NUTRITIVE VALUES PER SERVING:

FAT	FIBER	VIT. A	VIT. C	CAL	CAL FROM FAT
7.69gm	.34gm	470 IU	5.67mg	213	33%

CURRIED TURKEY AND BROCCOLI

Rice or pasta are nice accompaniments to this dish—include a bit of curry sauce on them, also.

1 tablespoon corn or safflower oil
1 tablespoon margarine or butter
1½ pounds turkey breast, sliced into ⅜-inch slices
2 medium onions, finely chopped
1 tablespoon curry powder
½ teaspoon salt
¼ teaspoon pepper
2 tablespoons unbleached white flour
1½ cups turkey or chicken stock
1 cup low-fat milk
5 tablespoons nonfat dry milk
3 small bunches broccoli (about 2 pounds), divided into florets

Heat oil and margarine over medium heat in a large skillet. Add enough turkey slices to sauté in one layer. Sauté 1 minute on each side (don't overcook). Remove cooked slices and repeat until all slices are cooked. Keep cooked turkey slices warm.

Add onions to pan and sauté for 5 minutes. Add curry powder, salt, pepper, and flour and blend with onions until golden brown, stirring constantly. Add stock and bring to a boil. Cook at a low boil for 5 minutes, stirring frequently.

Mix low-fat milk with nonfat dry milk and add to sauce. Bring to a boil, reduce heat, and simmer for 5 minutes or until sauce is smooth. While making sauce, steam broccoli until crisp-tender.

Return turkey slices to sauce and heat gently, moving slices around so each one is coated with sauce and heated through. To serve, place turkey in center of each plate and coat with sauce. Arrange broccoli around turkey, spooning some sauce over broccoli.

Serves 8

NUTRITIVE VALUES PER SERVING:

FAT	FIBER	VIT. A	VIT. C	CAL	CAL FROM FAT
8.98gm	9.95gm	4140 IU	144mg	277	29%

JAMBALAYA

3 tablespoons margarine or butter
$\frac{1}{2}$ cup chopped onion
$\frac{1}{2}$ cup chopped scallions
$\frac{1}{2}$ cup chopped green bell pepper
$\frac{1}{2}$ cup chopped celery
2 cloves garlic, minced
2 cups chicken broth
$1\frac{1}{2}$ cups chopped tomatoes
$\frac{1}{4}$ cup chopped fresh parsley
$\frac{1}{2}$ teaspoon salt
$\frac{1}{8}$ teaspoon pepper
$\frac{1}{4}$ teaspoon thyme
$\frac{1}{8}$ teaspoon cayenne pepper
1 bay leaf
1 cup brown rice, uncooked
8 halved boneless, skinless chicken breasts

Heat margarine over medium heat in a large pan. Add onion, scallions, green pepper, celery, and garlic. Sauté for five minutes.

Add chicken broth, tomatoes, parsley, salt, pepper, thyme, cayenne, and bay leaf. Cover and bring to a boil. Add rice and chicken and cook, covered, over medium-low heat for 45 minutes, stirring occasionally. Serve hot.

Serves 8

NUTRITIVE VALUES PER SERVING:

FAT	FIBER	VIT. A	VIT. C	CAL	CAL FROM FAT
7.86gm	3.69gm	992 IU	29.5mg	269	26%

MANDARIN ORANGE CHICKEN WITH BROCCOLI

3 tablespoons margarine or butter
¼ cup minced onion
¼ cup unbleached white flour
1 tablespoon paprika
½ teaspoon salt
¼ teaspoon pepper
8 chicken breast halves, boned and skinned
1 cup chicken broth
1 cup low-fat milk
1½ pounds broccoli, broken into florets, stems peeled and sliced
1 8-ounce can mandarin oranges, drained

Melt margarine in a large skillet. Sauté onions over medium heat until soft. Combine flour, paprika, salt, and pepper and coat chicken with flour mixture by shaking together in a bag, one chicken breast half at a time.

Add chicken to skillet and sauté 5 minutes on each side. Remove chicken from skillet; add broth and bring to a boil. Boil for 5 minutes to thicken a bit, stirring often. Add milk and simmer for 5 minutes, stirring often. Return chicken to skillet, baste with sauce, and simmer for 10 minutes on low heat, basting chicken again several times with the sauce.

Steam broccoli while chicken is simmering. To serve, surround chicken with broccoli. Spoon sauce over chicken and broccoli and garnish with mandarin oranges.

Serves 8

NUTRITIVE VALUES PER SERVING:

FAT	FIBER	VIT. A	VIT. C	CAL	CAL FROM FAT
7.91gm	5.42gm	2399 IU	81.6mg	226	32%

MUSTARD SAUCE TURKEY
WITH BRUSSELS SPROUTS

Small boiled potatoes tossed with chopped parsley are a good accompaniment to this dish.

$1\frac{1}{2}$ pounds turkey breast, cut into cubes
$1\frac{1}{2}$ cups chicken or turkey broth
3 cups brussels sprouts
5 teaspoons margarine or butter
1 cup chopped onion
$\frac{1}{4}$ cup white wine vinegar
$\frac{1}{2}$ cup water
1 teaspoon thyme
$\frac{1}{2}$ teaspoon salt
$\frac{1}{4}$ teaspoon pepper
2 cups low-fat milk
2 tablespoons dijon mustard
$\frac{1}{4}$ teaspoon cayenne pepper

Simmer turkey cubes in broth for 5–10 minutes, until tender. Steam sprouts until barely done.

Heat margarine in a large skillet and sauté onion for 10 minutes. Add vinegar, water, thyme, salt, and pepper and simmer over medium-low heat until most of the liquid evaporates, about 10 minutes. Stir in milk and bring to a boil, stirring. Simmer 10 more minutes or until thickened a bit, stirring often. Add mustard, cayenne, turkey cubes, and brussels sprouts and cook 5 minutes more to heat through.

Serves 6

NUTRITIVE VALUES PER SERVING:

FAT	FIBER	VIT. A	VIT. C	CAL	CAL FROM FAT
8.11gm	2.71gm	670 IU	70.8mg	239	31%

PERFECTLY POACHED CHICKEN

This method produces a tender and flavorful chicken, which may be eaten plain, sauced, or cut up for salads or sandwiches.

1 fresh whole chicken (or 1 fresh whole turkey breast)
2 scallions, sliced into a few pieces
2 slices fresh ginger (optional)
Enough water to cover chicken

Remove fat and skin from chicken; rinse. Bring water to a boil in a large pot; add scallions, ginger, and chicken to the boiling water (boiling water seals flavor and juices into the chicken). When water comes back to a boil, skim surface, cover pot, and turn off heat. Don't remove from burner or lift cover.

After 1 hour, lift out chicken and place in ice water (this step also seals juices into the chicken). After 15 minutes, remove chicken from ice water and drain. Use immediately or refrigerate.

Serves 4

NUTRITIVE VALUES PER SERVING:

WITH WHOLE CHICKEN:

FAT	FIBER	VIT. A	VIT. C	CAL	CAL FROM FAT
8.47gm	.74gm	535 IU	7.6mg	224	34%

WITH WHOLE TURKEY BREAST:

FAT	FIBER	VIT. A	VIT. C	CAL	CAL FROM FAT
3.66gm	.23gm	150 IU	2.4mg	180	18%

SPICY SESAME NOODLES WITH TURKEY AND SCALLOPS

¼ cup sesame seeds

½ pound fresh scallops

3 tablespoons rice wine vinegar

2 tablespoons peanut butter

1½ tablespoons honey

¾ teaspoon dijon mustard

2½ tablespoons soy sauce

1 teaspoon Chinese chili oil (found in Oriental section of market)

2 tablespoons Chinese sesame oil (found in Oriental section of market)

3 tablespoons chicken or turkey broth

1½ tablespoons orange juice

1 pound boneless, cooked turkey white meat, cut into bite-sized pieces (boneless, cooked chicken breast may be substituted)

1 cup grated carrots

½ pound whole-wheat vermicelli

½ cup chopped scallions

Toast sesame seeds by heating on medium heat for 5 minutes in an ungreased frying pan, tossing several times.

To poach scallops, place in simmering water and simmer for a few minutes, just until done (scallops are done when they turn opaque).

Make sauce by mixing vinegar, peanut butter, honey, mustard, soy sauce, oils, broth, and orange juice. Marinate scallops, cooked turkey, and carrots in half the sauce for at least 1 hour. Cook vermicelli, drain well, and toss with remaining half of the sauce. Heat gently over low heat while also heating turkey mixture, separately, over low heat.

To serve, arrange noodles in the center of a large platter, surround with the turkey mixture, and sprinkle with sesame seeds and scallions. Serve immediately.

Serves 8

NUTRITIVE VALUES PER SERVING:

FAT	FIBER	VIT. A	VIT. C	CAL	CAL FROM FAT
11.0gm	2.56gm	3154 IU	5.46mg	339	29%

SWEET AND SOUR CHICKEN WITH VEGETABLES

2 cups raw brown rice
3 tablespoons corn or safflower oil
1½ cups coarsely chopped onion
2 large carrots, sliced
2 stalks celery, sliced
1½ cups coarsely chopped green bell pepper
2 cups tomato sauce
½ cup water
¼ cup brown sugar
2 tablespoons fresh lemon juice
1 20-ounce can pineapple chunks, in juice, drained
2 cups cooked chicken cubes
1 16-ounce block tofu (soybean curd), drained

Start cooking rice about 20 minutes before beginning chicken and vegetables.

Heat oil and sauté vegetables until tender-crisp. Stir in tomato sauce, water, brown sugar, lemon juice, pineapple chunks, and chicken and simmer 10 minutes. Cut tofu into 1-inch cubes and add to sauce. Cover and cook on low heat for 5 minutes, stirring gently. Serve over hot rice.

Serves 6

NUTRITIVE VALUES PER SERVING:

FAT	FIBER	VIT. A	VIT. C	CAL	CAL FROM FAT
13.7gm	9.86gm	3751 IU	80.2mg	571	22%

TURKEY BREAST WITH LEMON AND CAULIFLOWER

1 cup raw brown rice
2 cups chicken or turkey broth
1½ pounds boneless turkey breast, skin
    removed, cut into bite-sized pieces
1 large cauliflower (about 2 pounds), broken
    into florets
3 tablespoons margarine or butter
4 tablespoons unbleached white flour
2 cups low-fat milk
¼ cup fresh lemon juice
½ teaspoon thyme
½ teaspoon salt
½ teaspoon pepper
1 cup chopped fresh parsley
Paprika

Start rice when beginning recipe, cooking according to package directions. Keep warm if done before recipe is completed.

Heat broth to a boil and add turkey pieces. Bring to a simmer and cook 5 minutes or until done. Drain.

Steam cauliflower for 5–10 minutes, or until done, while beginning sauce. Keep cauliflower warm.

Melt margarine; add flour and stir until golden brown. Add milk and bring to a boil, whisking and cooking over medium heat until thickened. Still whisking, add lemon juice, thyme, salt, and pepper and combine. Add cooked turkey pieces and heat through.

To serve, place rice in center of platter. Surround with cauliflower. Pour turkey mixture over rice, drizzling some sauce over cauliflower. Decorate with chopped parsley and sprinkle with paprika.

Serves 6

NUTRITIVE VALUES PER SERVING:

FAT	FIBER	VIT. A	VIT. C	CAL	CAL FROM FAT
11.5gm	4.80gm	1292 IU	68.6mg	386	27%

TURKEY CHILI WITH GARNISHES

1 pound cooked turkey breast, cut into small
   cubes
4 cloves garlic, minced
2 tablespoons corn or safflower oil
1 cup chopped green bell pepper
1 cup chopped onion
½ teaspoon celery seed
¼ teaspoon cayenne pepper
1 teaspoon ground cumin
2 bay leaves
2 tablespoons chili powder
1 teaspoon oregano
½ teaspoon salt
2 15-ounce cans tomato sauce
2 15-ounce cans kidney beans, drained

GARNISHES

¾ cup chopped fresh cilantro (coriander)
½ cup chopped onion
¾ cup low-fat yogurt
¾ cup grated part-skim mozzarella cheese
1 recipe baked Tortilla Chips (see Index)

In a 3-quart pan, sauté turkey cubes and garlic in oil for 5 minutes over medium heat. Add the green pepper and onion and cook on low heat for 10 minutes. Add the seasonings; stir to coat turkey and vegetables.

Add tomato sauce and beans; stir. Cook 1 hour, uncovered. Serve chili in individual dishes with bowls of garnishes in the center of the table.

Serves 6

NUTRITIVE VALUES PER SERVING:

FAT	FIBER	VIT. A	VIT. C	CAL	CAL FROM FAT
12.1gm	13.4gm	2361 IU	74.3mg	453	24%

CORNED BEEF (without nitrates)

Even though this corned beef is easy and quick to prepare, don't plan on serving it until it has cured in the pickling spices for at least 2 weeks.

TO CURE MEAT:

¾ cup kosher (coarse) salt

2 tablespoons brown sugar

3 tablespoons pickling spice

4 bay leaves

1 tablespoon cream of tartar

5 cloves garlic, sliced

1 medium onion, sliced

1 6- to 7-pound lean beef roast (preferably round), trimmed of all fat

In a bowl, combine all ingredients except the roast, and gently toss. Rub mixture into all surfaces of the roast. Set roast into a bag that can be closed airtight ("zip" closures are good for this). Pat any remaining spice mixture onto the meat in the bag. Close bag, squeezing out as much air as possible. Place into a large bowl or pan and cover with a plate and a weight—a dinner plate and a brick will do.

Leave roast in the refrigerator for 2 weeks and up to a month. If the bag breaks or leaks, repackage roast with all spices in a new bag. Turn the bag over daily, massaging spices into meat.

TO COOK MEAT:

1 6- to 7-pound lean corned beef roast, trimmed of all fat

1 carrot per person

1 rib of celery per person

1 small onion per person

½ rutabaga or turnip per person

1 medium potato per person

⅛ head cabbage per person

Rinse meat well and soak it in water for several hours, changing water often to get rid of excess salt. Place meat in a large kettle filled with enough cold water to cover meat by 2 or 3 inches. Bring to a boil; skim off any foam, and simmer for about 3½ hours, partially covered, until meat is tender when pierced with a fork. Add vegetables during the last 30 minutes.

Leftovers make a delicious hash, and freeze well if packaged properly. We also like to serve corned beef with 2 or 3 kinds of mustard and flavorful whole-grain breads, such as rye and pumpernickel.

*Makes 24 3-ounce servings**

---

*By the time the roast has been cured and cooked, a 6-pound roast will yield approximately 24 3-ounce servings.

NUTRITIVE VALUES PER SERVING:

FAT	FIBER	VIT. A	VIT. C	CAL	CAL FROM FAT
8.62gm	16.2gm	8332 IU	89.6mg	409	19%

COUNTRY SAUSAGE AND POTATOES

This is an ideal dish for brunch or a light supper.

4 medium potatoes, unpeeled
1 pound lean pork, all visible fat removed, ground
1 tablespoon corn or safflower oil
1 cup chopped onions
1½ teaspoons poultry seasoning
½ teaspoon salt
¼ teaspoon pepper
1 cup chopped parsley

Cut potatoes into small cubes and steam for 5 minutes, or until almost tender. Drain. Grind pork in food processor, or have your butcher do this for you. (The ground pork found in the meat section of a market is too high in fat.)

In a nonstick pan, cook ground pork (without any added oil) until crumbly. Drain off any fat and set meat aside.

Clean pan and return to heat. Add oil; sauté onions over medium heat with poultry seasoning, salt, and pepper until onions are soft. Add steamed potatoes and cook over low heat for 15 minutes. Add pork and cook, stirring gently, for 15 minutes more. Sprinkle with parsley and serve immediately.

Serves 6

NUTRITIVE VALUES PER SERVING:

FAT	FIBER	VIT. A	VIT. C	CAL	CAL FROM FAT
10.1gm	5.19gm	858 IU	46.2mg	289	32%*

*With the pork fat drained off, the percentage of calories from fat is even less than this analysis indicates.

CREOLE SAUSAGE WITH RICE AND BEANS

CREOLE SAUSAGE MIXTURE*

1 pound lean pork, all visible fat removed, ground
⅓ cup finely chopped onion
1 clove garlic, minced
½ teaspoon salt
¼ teaspoon pepper
¼ teaspoon cayenne pepper
¼ teaspoon paprika
½ cup parsley, chopped
⅛ teaspoon allspice

VEGETABLE MIXTURE

2 tablespoons corn or vegetable oil
1¼ cup chopped onions
2 cloves garlic, minced
1 tablespoon chili powder
¼ teaspoon basil
¼ teaspoon oregano
¼ teaspoon ground cumin
2 cups chopped cabbage
1 cup grated carrots
3 cups chopped tomatoes
2 16-ounce cans kidney beans, drained
1 cup uncooked brown rice
1 cup chicken (or other) broth

Grind pork in food processor, or have your butcher do this for you. (The ground pork found in the meat section of a market is too high in fat.) Mix ground pork with remaining sausage ingredients. In a large saucepan, cook sausage mixture (without added fat) until crumbly and thoroughly cooked. Drain off all fat.

In a clean pan, heat oil and sauté onions, garlic, and spices for 5 minutes over medium-high heat. Add cabbage and carrots and cook 5 minutes. Add tomatoes, drained beans, rice, broth, and cooked sausage meat and bring to a boil. Reduce heat, cover, and cook over low heat for 1 hour. More broth may be added if mixture seems dry. Remove cover, raise heat to medium, and cook 15 minutes more. Serve hot.

Serves 8

---

*If just the Creole sausages are desired, form sausage mixture into 6 oblongs or patties and bake, broil, or cook in nonstick pan.

NUTRITIVE VALUES PER SERVING:

FAT	FIBER	VIT. A	VIT. C	CAL	CAL FROM FAT
10.5gm	14.5gm	3277 IU	41.2mg	366	26%

FRENCH BEEF WITH VEGETABLES

2 pounds boneless beef roast, weighed with all
 fat removed
8 medium carrots, quartered
8 medium potatoes, quartered
1 large onion, sliced
2 cloves garlic, minced
1 teaspoon thyme
½ teaspoon salt
¼ teaspoon pepper
½ cup red wine
2 tablespoons margarine or butter, softened
2 tablespoons flour
1 cup chopped parsley

Preheat oven to 250°F. Place roast in a large casserole with a cover. Arrange carrots, potatoes, and onion around and over roast. Sprinkle meat and vegetables with garlic, thyme, salt, and pepper. Pour wine over meat and vegetables. Roast, covered, at 250°F for 4½ hours.

Remove roast and vegetables. Place roast, sliced or unsliced, on a platter and surround with vegetables. Keep warm.

Heat juices in casserole over high heat. Combine margarine and flour into a paste and stir into the bubbling liquid. Boil for a few minutes until thickened, whisking constantly. Pour a bit of sauce over meat and vegetables on platter and sprinkle with parsley. Pass remaining sauce.

Makes 8 3-ounce servings

NUTRITIVE VALUES PER SERVING:

FAT	FIBER	VIT. A	VIT. C	CAL	CAL FROM FAT
10.6gm	8.69gm	8516 IU	44.7mg	371	26%

FRENCH VEAL RAGOUT

Served with a green salad and crusty wheat bread, this would make an easy and delicious buffet dinner.

2 pounds lean veal, cut into small cubes
1 cup tomato sauce
5 carrots, sliced
1 cup chopped onions
2 cups chopped tomatoes
⅓ cup water
⅓ cup white wine
1 cup chopped cabbage
1 cup chopped rutabagas or turnips
¾ teaspoon salt
½ teaspoon pepper
2 cups chopped unpeeled potatoes
2 cups chopped fresh parsley

Preheat oven to 250°F. Mix all ingredients thoroughly in a heavy casserole with a cover. Bake, covered, for 5 hours at 250°F without removing cover during cooking process. Stir well; sprinkle with parsley and serve.

Serves 10

NUTRITIVE VALUES PER SERVING:

FAT	FIBER	VIT. A	VIT. C	CAL	CAL FROM FAT
7.4gm	5.66gm	5846 IU	53.0mg	217	31%

GREEK MEATBALLS

4 ounces bulgur (cracked wheat)
1 cup water
1 pound lean lamb, all visible fat removed,
    ground
2 eggs, beaten
¾ cup minced onion
¼ teaspoon cinnamon
½ teaspoon salt
½ teaspoon pepper
2 teaspoons fresh lemon juice
2 teaspoons honey
2 tablespoons dried mint
⅓ cup sliced almonds
1½ cups chopped fresh parsley

MINT SAUCE

1 tablespoon dried mint
1 cup low-fat yogurt
2 tablespoons fresh lemon juice
½ teaspoon salt
1 clove garlic, minced

Soak bulgur for 1 hour in 1 cup water. Drain bulgur well and combine thoroughly with ground lamb. Add eggs and combine well. Add onion, cinnamon, salt, pepper, lemon juice, honey, mint, and almonds. Thoroughly combine all ingredients.

Form into 32 meatballs. In a nonstick skillet, cook meatballs over medium heat until browned, tossing often—about 10 minutes. Unless the pan is very large, the meatballs will probably need to be browned in 2 batches. Keep browned meatballs warm while making sauce.

Drain any excess fat from pan and turn heat to low. Combine mint, yogurt, lemon juice, salt, and garlic to make Mint Sauce. Add Mint Sauce and meatballs to pan and cook together on low heat for about 15 minutes, stirring gently so the meatballs do not break. Serve hot, sprinkled with parsley.

Serves 8

NUTRITIVE VALUES PER SERVING:

FAT	FIBER	VIT. A	VIT. C	CAL	CAL FROM FAT
9.58gm	6.85gm	1040 IU	23.2mg	336	26%

ITALIAN SAUSAGES

These make wonderful sandwiches—serve on crusty wheat rolls with lightly sautéed green peppers and onions. They are also especially good with whole-wheat spaghetti and Marinara Sauce (see Index).

1 pound lean ground round
½ pound lean ground veal
¼ cup wheat germ
½ cup evaporated skim milk
3 tablespoons dried minced onions
2 teaspoons poultry seasoning
1½ teaspoons garlic salt
1½ teaspoons oregano
1½ teaspoons fennel seeds
1 teaspoon red pepper flakes for "hot" sausages;
 ½ teaspoon or less for "mild"

Combine all ingredients and mix thoroughly. Shape into 8 oblong sausage shapes. Broil, bake, or cook in nonstick pan.

Serves 8

NUTRITIVE VALUES PER SERVING:

FAT	FIBER	VIT. A	VIT. C	CAL	CAL FROM FAT
9.36gm	4.79gm	238 IU	51.9mg	341	25%

MEXICAN-STYLE BEEF STEW

2 pounds beef round, weighed with all fat
   removed, cut into small cubes
1 cup chopped onion
2 cloves garlic, minced
1 cup chopped green bell pepper
1 cup tomato sauce
1 tablespoon red wine vinegar
1 teaspoon oregano
½ teaspoon salt
2 tablespoons diced mild green chilies (canned)
2 tablespoons unbleached white flour
3 cups raw brown rice (about 9 cups cooked)
2½ cups chopped fresh parsley

In a heavy pot with a cover, mix all ingredients except rice and parsley. Simmer over low heat for 2 hours, covered, stirring every half hour. After stew has cooked for about 1 hour, start rice, cooking according to package directions. Serve stew over hot rice, sprinkling each serving with parsley.

Serves 10

NUTRITIVE VALUES PER SERVING:

FAT	FIBER	VIT. A	VIT. C	CAL	CAL FROM FAT
5.07gm	4.64gm	1605 IU	52.1mg	281	16%

OVEN-ROASTED LAMB WITH VEGETABLE SAUCE

2 pounds boneless lamb roast, weighed with all
visible fat removed

½ teaspoon salt

¼ teaspoon pepper

2-3 lamb bones (if available), all visible fat
removed

3 carrots, coarsely chopped

2 cloves garlic, sliced

1 large onion

3 whole cloves

3 tablespoons olive oil

1 additional garlic clove

½ teaspoon thyme

½ teaspoon salt

¼ teaspoon pepper

1 bay leaf

2 tomatoes, peeled, seeded, and chopped (to
peel and seed, see Chilled Fresh Tomato
Soup)

½ cup red wine

½ cup chopped fresh parsley

10 cups cooked white beans, cooked according
to package directions

Preheat oven to 400°F. Rub lamb with salt and pepper and arrange on rack in roasting pan. Surround with bones, carrots, sliced garlic cloves, and the onion stuck with 3 cloves. Pour olive oil over bones and vegetables and roast at 400°F for 30 minutes. Reduce heat to 350°F and roast 30 minutes more.

Transfer lamb to a casserole with a cover and add remaining garlic clove, thyme, salt, pepper, bay leaf, and tomatoes. Add bones and vegetables from roasting pan. Add wine to roasting pan, stirring to incorporate any browned bits into the wine, and pour over lamb in casserole. Cover tightly and cook at 225°F for 5 hours.

Transfer lamb to a hot platter and remove any strings. Keep warm. Discard bones, bay leaf, and the cloves from the onion. Skim off any fat, leaving sauce and vegetables in casserole. Over medium-high heat, boil pan juices in casserole for a few minutes, mashing vegetables into the sauce. Sprinkle sauce with chopped parsley and serve with the lamb. Accompany with cooked white beans, with some of the sauce spooned over beans.

Serves 10

NUTRITIVE VALUES PER SERVING:

FAT	FIBER	VIT. A	VIT. C	CAL	CAL FROM FAT
12.0gm	16.4gm	2902 IU	13.6mg	432	25%

PORTUGUESE CABBAGE ROLLS

1 head cabbage
1 tablespoon margarine
1 tablespoon broth, fat removed
1 cup grated carrots
1 cup onion, chopped
1 pound lean ground round
2 cups cooked brown rice
$\frac{1}{2}$ teaspoon salt
$\frac{1}{4}$ teaspoon pepper
$\frac{1}{2}$ teaspoon oregano
$\frac{1}{2}$ teaspoon thyme
1 tablespoon fresh lemon juice
1 28-ounce can tomatoes, drained and coarsely
    chopped
2 cups beef broth

Core cabbage, leaving head intact. Place in large kettle of boiling water. Cook, partly covered, for 10 minutes. Lift out carefully and drain. Remove 16–20 outer leaves and dry gently.

Melt margarine with broth; sauté carrots and onions for 5 minutes. Add meat, rice, seasonings, and lemon juice. Cook for about 10 minutes, breaking up meat, until meat is thoroughly cooked.

Carefully trim thick center rib from each cabbage leaf to facilitate rolling. Place 3–4 tablespoons meat mixture in center of each leaf and roll leaves up and around filling, tucking in ends. Cabbage rolls may be tied with thread or secured with toothpicks. Place rolls, seam side down, in a 9" × 13" pan. Pour tomatoes and broth over rolls. Cover and bake in a preheated 375°F oven for 1 hour. Remove cover and bake for 30 minutes more, basting frequently with juice. If cabbage rolls start to brown, lay a piece of foil lightly over them. Serve with sauce.

If a thicker sauce is desired, transfer sauce to a saucepan, keeping cabbage rolls warm in oven. Add 2 tablespoons cornstarch mixed with 2 tablespoons water to the boiling sauce, and whisk until thickened.

Serves 8

NUTRITIVE VALUES PER SERVING:

FAT	FIBER	VIT. A	VIT. C	CAL	CAL FROM FAT
6.81gm	5.11gm	4062 IU	43.6mg	213	29%

RAGOUT OF LAMB

2 pounds boneless lamb, weighed with all fat removed

1 tablespoon olive oil

1 tablespoon margarine

2 cups chopped onions

1 6-ounce can tomato paste

3 cups chopped tomatoes

1 bay leaf

½ teaspoon salt

½ teaspoon pepper

½ teaspoon ground coriander

1 teaspoon sugar

1 cup red wine

9 cups cooked brown rice (about 3 cups uncooked)

Cut lamb into small cubes. Heat oil and margarine in a heavy saucepan. When hot, cook lamb over medium-high heat until all pieces are browned.

Push meat aside and cook onions until tender, but not browned. Add tomato paste, chopped tomatoes, bay leaf, salt, pepper, coriander, sugar, and wine. Stir until blended. Turn heat down and simmer, covered, for 2–2½ hours, stirring occasionally until tender. About 1 hour before ragout is done, start rice, cooking according to package directions.

Serve ragout over hot rice.

Serves 10

NUTRITIVE VALUES PER SERVING:

FAT	FIBER	VIT. A	VIT. C	CAL	CAL FROM FAT
11.3gm	5.58gm	1127 IU	16.0mg	422	24%

SAUSAGE AND PEPPERS ITALIANO

2¾ cups raw brown rice
1 recipe Italian Sausages (see Index)
4 cups coarsely chopped green bell pepper
2 cups coarsely chopped onion
2 cloves garlic, minced
¼ cup dry white wine
¼ cup water
1 cup tomato sauce
1 teaspoon oregano
1 large tomato, chopped

Start rice, cooking according to package directions. Shape Italian Sausage mixture into 24 meatballs. Brown meatballs over medium heat with no extra fat, turning frequently to brown all over. Remove meatballs with a slotted spoon and set aside.

Add peppers, onion, garlic, wine, and water to pan and cook, uncovered, for 5 minutes on medium-high heat. Return meatballs to pan. Add tomato sauce, oregano, and tomato. Cover and simmer for 10 minutes. Uncover and simmer until sauce is thickened a bit, stirring gently. Serve over hot brown rice.

Serves 8

NUTRITIVE VALUES PER SERVING:

FAT	FIBER	VIT. A	VIT. C	CAL	CAL FROM FAT
8.91gm	6.77gm	831 IU	108mg	429	19%

SOUTH AMERICAN
CHILI BEEF IN TORTILLAS

1 cup chopped onion

2 cloves garlic, minced

1 tablespoon corn or safflower oil

2 pounds beef round with all fat removed, cut
into small cubes

2 tablespoons flour

1 cup chopped green bell pepper

1 cup tomato sauce

2 tablespoons red wine vinegar

1 teaspoon ground cumin

1 teaspoon oregano

½ teaspoon salt

3 tablespoons diced mild chilies (canned)

10 large whole-wheat flour tortillas (white may
be substituted)

2½ cups shredded lettuce

Sauté onion and garlic in oil, until onions are soft. Add beef
cubes and sauté over medium-high heat for 5 minutes. Add flour
and toss with beef cubes and onions to coat. Add all remaining
ingredients except tortillas and lettuce and mix gently but
thoroughly.

Simmer 2½ hours on medium heat, covered, stirring every half
hour. Uncover and cook for another half hour to thicken sauce
slightly. When beef is tender and ready to serve, heat flour
tortillas until warm but not crisp. Fill each warm tortilla with ⅟₁₀
the beef and ¼ cup shredded lettuce and roll up.

Serves 10

Nutritive Values per Serving:

FAT	FIBER	VIT. A	VIT. C	CAL	CAL FROM FAT
8.69gm	1.52gm	467 IU	28.2mg	264	30%

SOUTHERN BEEF LOAF

1½ pounds very lean ground round
1 egg, slightly beaten
¾ cup sweetened applesauce
¾ cup dry bread crumbs
1 cup finely chopped onion
1 cup finely chopped celery
1 cup finely chopped carrots
¾ cup very finely chopped green bell pepper
1 clove garlic, minced
½ cup tomato juice
¼ teaspoon salt
¼ teaspoon pepper

Soften beef in a large bowl by mixing with fork. Mix egg and applesauce and thoroughly combine with beef. Add bread crumbs and mix well with beef mixture.

Add vegetables, tomato juice, salt, and pepper to beef mixture and mix thoroughly. Press into loaf pan, smooth top, and bake in a preheated 350°F oven for 45 minutes. Drain off any fat and bake for 45 minutes more. Let set for a few minutes before slicing.

Serves 8

NUTRITIVE VALUES PER SERVING:

FAT	FIBER	VIT. A	VIT. C	CAL	CAL FROM FAT
8.02gm	2.66gm	2292 IU	25.8mg	215	34%

SPINACH-STUFFED FLANK STEAK

1 1½-pound beef flank steak
1½ tablespoons dijon mustard
2 scallions, sliced
2 packages frozen chopped spinach, thawed and
    squeezed dry
½ cup bread crumbs
½ cup chopped fresh parsley
½ teaspoon oregano
½ teaspoon basil
⅛ teaspoon pepper
1 clove garlic, minced
2 teaspoons olive oil
4 teaspoons beef broth, fat removed
1½ cups beef broth, fat removed

Spread steak flat. Cut in half horizontally, starting at the tapered side (not end) and stopping within ½ inch of the wide side. Open steak out flat and cover with mustard.

Combine scallions, spinach, bread crumbs, parsley, oregano, basil, pepper, and garlic, and spread the mixture evenly over the opened steak. Roll up, jelly roll style, starting with one of the tapered sides so the steak keeps its original length. Tie the rolled roast with string.

Heat olive oil and 4 teaspoons broth in a casserole with a cover, and brown meat on all sides. Add 1½ cups broth, cover, and bake for 2 hours at 350°F. Cut into 6–8 slices and serve with any liquid from the pan.

Serves 6–8

NUTRITIVE VALUES PER SERVING:

FAT	FIBER	VIT. A	VIT. C	CAL	CAL FROM FAT
6.34gm	5.35gm	7231 IU	20.6mg	194	29%

STUFFED PEPPERS CALIFORNIA

1 pound lean ground round
1½ cups cooked brown rice
1 egg, beaten
½ cup grated carrots
½ teaspoon salt
½ teaspoon pepper
1 teaspoon oregano
8 medium green bell peppers
2 cups chopped tomatoes
1 cup tomato sauce
½ cup finely chopped onion
1 tablespoon fresh lemon juice

Combine ground beef, rice, egg, carrots, salt, pepper, and oregano and mix well. Cut green peppers in half lengthwise and remove membranes and seeds. Lightly stuff pepper halves with meat mixture. Place peppers in a baking dish that holds them securely without crowding.

Combine tomatoes, tomato sauce, onion, and lemon juice. Spoon over and around peppers. Cover dish tightly with foil and bake in a preheated 350°F oven for 1 hour. Serve immediately.

Serves 8

NUTRITIVE VALUES PER SERVING:

FAT	FIBER	VIT. A	VIT. C	CAL	CAL FROM FAT
6.02gm	4.15gm	2668 IU	163mg	189	29%

VEAL CHORIZO

Serve these sausages alone, in Marinara Sauce (see Index) over pasta, or on crusty wheat rolls, as sandwiches.

1 pound lean beef round, all visible fat removed, ground

1 pound lean pork, all visible fat removed, ground

1 pound lean veal, all visible fat removed, ground

1 cup onion, chopped

3 cloves garlic, minced

½ cup evaporated skim milk

1 tablespoon chili powder

1 tablespoon paprika

2 teaspoons oregano

1 teaspoon ground cumin

1 teaspoon ground coriander

¼ teaspoon Tabasco sauce

1 tablespoon red wine vinegar

1 teaspoon salt

½ teaspoon pepper

Place all ingredients in a bowl and combine thoroughly. Shape into 16 sausage patties or oblongs, and bake, broil, or cook in a nonstick pan.

These sausages will freeze well, either cooked or uncooked.

Makes 16 3-ounce sausages

NUTRITIVE VALUES PER SERVING:

FAT	FIBER	VIT. A	VIT. C	CAL	CAL FROM FAT
9.55gm	3.63gm	42.2 IU	1.16mg	313	27%

VEAL-RICE STROGANOFF

1½ pounds veal, all fat removed, cut into small
   cubes
1 tablespoon broth, fat removed
1 tablespoon corn or safflower oil
½ cup chopped onion
1 garlic clove, minced
½ teaspoon salt
¼ teaspoon pepper
1 teaspoon paprika
3½ cups beef broth
1 cup uncooked brown rice
½ cup low-fat yogurt
½ cup chopped fresh parsley

Brown veal cubes in the 1 tablespoon broth and 1 tablespoon oil;
add onion; cook 3 minutes. Add garlic, salt, pepper, and paprika
and cook 5 more minutes. Add beef broth and rice and bring to
a boil. Reduce heat and simmer, covered, for 30 minutes. Stir.
Simmer 15 minutes more.

Remove from heat and slowly add yogurt. Return to heat and
cook on lowest heat for 15 minutes. Sprinkle with parsley before
serving.

Serves 8

NUTRITIVE VALUES PER SERVING:

FAT	FIBER	VIT. A	VIT. C	CAL	CAL FROM FAT
9.30gm	2.05gm	332 IU	7.61mg	248	34%

VEAL ROAST ROYALE

1 tablespoon margarine or butter
1 tablespoon corn or safflower oil
1 3-pound veal roast, boned and tied, weighed
 with all visible fat removed
2 carrots, chopped
2 onions, chopped
1 stalk celery, chopped
6 parsley sprigs
$\frac{1}{2}$ teaspoon thyme
$\frac{1}{2}$ teaspoon salt
$\frac{1}{4}$ teaspoon pepper
12 medium potatoes, halved
12 medium carrots, halved

Melt margarine and oil in a large ovenproof casserole with lid. Brown veal on all sides over medium heat. Remove veal when browned (about 15–20 minutes). Add chopped carrots, onions, and celery and all seasonings. Cook over low heat for 5 minutes. Return veal to casserole, surround with halved potatoes and carrots, and spoon margarine-vegetable mixture over meat, potatoes, and carrots, Cover casserole and bake in a preheated 325°F oven for 3½ hours. Baste and turn roast every half hour.

Remove roast and halved potatoes and halved carrots to serving platter and discard strings. Skim fat off sauce and place casserole over medium-high heat. Mash vegetables into liquid. Scrape the bottom and sides of the pan to incorporate any browned bits into sauce. Spoon some sauce over roast and pass the rest of the sauce.

Makes 12 3-ounce servings

NUTRITIVE VALUES PER SERVING:

FAT	FIBER	VIT. A	VIT. C	CAL	CAL FROM FAT
13.7gm	9.18gm	9483 IU	39.7mg	397	31%

VEAL STROGANOFF MADEIRA

1 pound veal scaloppine, all visible fat removed
(thin slices boneless, skinless chicken or
turkey can be substituted)
1 tablespoon corn or safflower oil
1 tablespoon chicken broth
2 cloves garlic, minced
½ cup very thinly sliced onions
1½ tablespoons unbleached white flour
½ teaspoon paprika
½ teaspoon salt
½ teaspoon pepper
1 cup low-fat milk
12 ounces pasta (preferably flat noodle type)
⅔ cup low-fat yogurt
⅓ cup sour cream
2 tablespoons madeira wine

Sauté veal slices in oil and broth over medium heat until just done. Remove veal to a plate.

Reduce heat; add garlic and onions to pan and sauté, stirring constantly, until onions are soft, adding a bit more broth if needed. Blend flour, paprika, salt, and pepper and sprinkle over onion mixture, stirring to coat. Stir in milk and bring to a boil. Reduce heat and simmer, uncovered, for 10 minutes, stirring often.

While sauce is simmering, cook pasta. Drain and keep warm when done.

Off heat, add yogurt, sour cream, and madeira to sauce. Return to heat and heat slowly to prevent yogurt from curdling. Add veal slices along with any liquid on plate, and heat through. Serve over hot pasta, spooning some sauce over pasta.

Serves 6

NUTRITIVE VALUES PER SERVING:

FAT	FIBER	VIT. A	VIT. C	CAL	CAL FROM FAT
12.4gm	.851gm	199 IU	1.89mg	382	29%

VENETIAN LIVER

6 cups cooked brown rice
2 tablespoons olive oil
1 cup thinly sliced onions
1 garlic clove, minced
⅛ teaspoon powdered sage
1 pound calves liver, cut across into ¼" strips
½ teaspoon salt
½ teaspoon pepper
¼ cup white wine
¼ cup fresh chopped parsley

Cook rice according to package directions; keep warm while sautéing liver.

Heat oil in a heavy skillet. Add onions, garlic, and sage and sauté over medium heat for 10 minutes. Remove onions with slotted spoon, leaving oil in pan, and reserve onions.

Pat the liver strips dry and season with salt and pepper. Heat skillet again and sauté liver for 2–3 minutes, or until lightly browned. Add reserved onions and cook with liver for 2 minutes.

Remove liver and onions with slotted spoon and set aside. Pour wine into skillet and boil about 2 minutes, incorporating any browned bits into the sauce. Return liver to pan and stir to coat liver with sauce. Heat through. Sprinkle with parsley and serve with rice.

Serves 5

NUTRITIVE VALUES PER SERVING:

FAT	FIBER	VIT. A	VIT. C	CAL	CAL FROM FAT
15.3gm	5.21gm	16,205 IU	31.7mg	465	30%

5
Meatless Entrées

Brazilian Black Beans and Rice
Broccoli and Cauliflower Neapolitan
Broccoli-Noodle Casserole
Broccoli Quiche
Brussels Sprouts and Cheese Bake
California Baked Beans
Cheese and Noodle Pudding
Cheese and Spinach with Noodles
Cheesy Soybean Bake
Chili-Cheese Pie
Cottage Cheese Enchiladas with
  Green Sauce
Curried Indian-Style Vegetables
Eggplant Parmesan
Lasagna Pinwheels with Two Sauces
Manicotti

Meatless Cabbage Rolls
Mexican Rice Crust Pizza
Pasta Primavera
Pepper and Cheese Bake
Potato-Cabbage Casserole
Potato-Cheese Pancakes
South American Peppers and Cheese
South American Squash
Spaghetti Squash and Rice Quiche
Spaghetti with Spinach and Mushrooms
Spinach-Cheese Dumplings
Spinach-Cheese Pancakes
Vegetarian Chili Casserole
Vegetarian Lasagna

Meatless Entrées

One way to reduce fat in your daily diet is to limit the number of servings of meat, fish, and poultry. Carefully designed vegetarian dishes can provide all of your protein, vitamin, and mineral needs—and assure you of good health. Whole grains, peas, beans, lentils, and vegetables are the mainstay of these dishes. Besides the benefit of a low-fat content, vegetarian entrées also contain a good amount of dietary fiber. Low fat and high fiber—no wonder meatless meals are so exceptional on a cancer risk–reduction diet.

We realize that to many of you, the words *meat* and *meal* are synonymous. Be assured that there really *are* many delicious entrées made without meat, fish, or poultry. Because of their flavorful, rich taste and robust texture, they fulfill both your physical and psychological need for food: there is something delicious to both chew and taste. And these meals are usually cheaper—a plus for the cost-conscious consumer.

Our goal in this chapter is twofold: to provide existing vegetarians with some exciting new dishes, and to introduce to those confirmed meateaters the versatility and satisfaction of a good meatless entrée. This chapter was not written to try to convert you to vegetarianism—there are many good books already on the market dealing with this subject. We merely want you to have good recipe choices available if you decide to make a transition towards vegetarianism, or if you'd occasionally like to incorporate a meatless entrée into your diet.

Plunging into a dietary regime that includes only plant foods (pure vegetarian) can be nutritionally dangerous if you don't know what you're doing. Before undertaking such a change, you may want to talk to your doctor or a registered dietitian (R.D.). Minerals, calcium, magnesium, iron, zinc, and iodine, as well as vitamin B_{12} (only found in animal foods) need to be emphasized in menu planning. A vitamin B_{12} supplement, and fortified cereal or soy milk, are usually necessary for pure vegetarians.

On a lacto-ovo vegetarian diet (which includes plant foods, milk, other dairy products, and eggs), the risk of having a nutrient-deficient diet is minimal. However, on this diet, it is easy to eat foods that are just as high in fat, saturated fat, and cholesterol as meat is. Hard cheese and eggs are the biggest offenders. One hard-cooked egg contains 250 milligrams of cholesterol and has 64% calories from fat. Hard cheeses such as swiss, monterey jack, or cheddar contain about 73% calories from fat and 56 milligrams of cholesterol per two-ounce serving. The maximum daily intake for cholesterol recommended by the American Heart Association is 300 milligrams.

Many Americans eat good meatless meals without even realizing it. Some of these include manicotti (ricotta cheese with a grain), pizza (part-skim cheese with a grain crust), spanish rice and beans, macaroni and cheese, and bean burritos (beans and a corn or wheat tortilla).

Some of these ingredients are incomplete proteins (don't contain all essential amino acids) by themselves, but when eaten in certain combinations become complete protein sources (contribute all nine essential amino acids). See Appendix I for a simple chart on combining proteins to make "complete" proteins.

Many Italian dishes boast good protein without meat. Instead they use ricotta and mozzarella cheeses, which are nourishing and tend to be lower in fat per serving than meat protein sources. These meals are even better when made with whole-wheat pasta, and part-skim ricotta or mozzarella cheeses. If you have never delighted in whole-wheat spaghetti, lasagna, or other pastas of this type, you are missing a taste treat. They have more flavor and texture than white pasta, and since they are made with the whole grain of the wheat, they contain more vitamins and fiber. If you buy vegetable pastas such as spinach or beet, read the package label to find out exactly what is in them— sometimes they are just refined flour products colored with vegetable dye. Usually, the amounts of vegetable in these pastas are too insignificant to do much nutritionally.

Pasta has the reputation with the general public of being

"fattening." Actually, it isn't the pasta itself, but how you dress it up that adds extra fat and calories to your meal. You can take basic Italian pasta dishes, make a few adjustments and substitutions, and come up with great-tasting low-fat meals. A simple meatless entrée of this type is ricotta-stuffed whole-wheat pasta shells with Marinara Sauce. After baking, top with a tablespoon of grated parmesan and a tablespoon of coarsely shredded mozzarella and put under the broiler for a minute.

We used all whole-grain pastas in testing these recipes. Many supermarkets now carry these products. If yours doesn't, check your local health food store. Whole-wheat products are worth the little extra effort it takes to obtain them. You can always buy enough pasta for several months, storing extra boxes in a cool, dry cabinet.

One interesting pasta dish in this chapter is Lasagna Pinwheels with Two Sauces. It has a creamy texture, using ricotta, cottage, and parmesan cheeses combined with chopped spinach and spices as the filling. It is served with Marinara Sauce around the edges, and topped with Light White Sauce for contrast. Serve with a salad of piquant greens such as chicory and endive, tossed with a hearty vinaigrette dressing.

Other pasta dishes include Spaghetti with Spinach and Mushrooms, Broccoli and Cauliflower Neapolitan, Manicotti, and Pasta Primavera.

Another popular combination that offers complete protein is rice and beans. Combining these two food staples has kept many civilizations healthy and thriving throughout the centuries. Brazilian Black Beans and Rice, Vegetarian Chili Casserole, and Mexican Rice Crust Pizza are a few of the dishes in this chapter that use this tasty combination.

We prefer to use brown rice in our recipes (see Chapter 7, Pasta, Rice, Grains, and Breads), mainly because it contributes about three times more dietary fiber than white rice and contains more vitamins and minerals. However, you can substitute the white variety in all of the rice recipes that follow. It is important to cook both rice and beans properly, or they will get mushy (see "Cooking Methods" at the end of this chapter introduction).

Quiche is still a favorite for brunch or a light supper. We have a wonderful Broccoli Quiche in which we mix cottage cheese and mozzarella together. Combine these ingredients with chopped parsley, spices, broccoli, a little flour, and two beaten eggs (most quiche recipes call for four to six eggs, adding too much fat and cholesterol to your meal). Then top the "pie" with seasoned bread crumbs before baking. It has all the taste and texture of quiche without a high amount of fat.

Potato-Cheese Pancakes is another exceptional brunch dish. Potatoes, carrots, low-fat cheese, and eggs give you protein and hearty flavor for a satisfying but light meal. Serve these pancakes with low-fat plain yogurt.

Two lovely "company" meals are Vegetarian Lasagna and South American Squash. The second dish is a delightful combination of sweet butternut squash, corn, grated mozzarella and cheddar cheeses, eggs, and piquant spices like chili powder, ground coriander, and cayenne pepper. It not only tastes delicious, but looks beautiful.

Curried Indian-Style Vegetables contains a wealth of vitamin- and fiber-rich foods found in typical Indian cuisine. It is a perfect dinner on a chilly winter night. Carrots, onions, potatoes, tomatoes, and cauliflower blend with garbanzo beans and herbs for a delicately spicy meal. Serve over rice with chopped green bell pepper and cucumber garnishes.

Potato-Cabbage Casserole combines two compatible ingredients with a creamy yogurt and sour cream sauce. This dish is absolutely scrumptious. You will find, as with other cabbage recipes in the book, that this often-disdained vegetable has a savory sweetness all its own. And when combined with potatoes and a creamy sauce, its flavor becomes even more buttery and mellow.

There are many more tasty and varied recipes in this chapter. We have randomly highlighted some of them to show how healthful ingredients make good-tasting meatless entrées. We are sure you will discover your own favorites.

Experience and enjoy these vegetarian meals as part of a personal good health plan, as well as a culinary delight.

COOKING METHODS
Brown Rice

Place 1¾ cups of cold water and 1 cup of rice into a saucepan. Cover tightly and bring to a boil. When mixture boils, reduce heat to low and simmer gently for 40 minutes. Remove from heat and fluff with a fork. This yields about 3 cups.

White Rice

Follow the same directions as above, except use 1½ cups of water and 1 cup of rice. Simmer for 20 minutes. This yields about 3 cups.

Beans

Wash by running under cool water. Soak, in enough water to cover, overnight. To cook, place beans in a large saucepan with enough fresh, cold water to cover and bring to a boil. When mixture reaches boiling point, lower heat and cook gently until tender. Cooking time will vary from 1 to 2½ hours depending on the size of the beans.

BRAZILIAN BLACK BEANS AND RICE

1 pound dried black beans
3 cups cooked brown rice (about 1 cup raw)
1 tablespoon corn or safflower oil
1 cup chopped onion
3 garlic cloves, minced
½ teaspoon salt
⅛ teaspoon pepper
1 tablespoon olive oil
1 tablespoon red wine vinegar
Garnishes: chopped onion, salsa, avocado or guacamole, fresh coriander, yogurt, baked Tortilla Chips (see Index)

Soak the beans overnight in enough water to cover. Drain off water and place beans in a pot with just enough water to cover beans. Cook over low heat for 2 hours or until beans are tender. Drain.

Start rice, cooking according to package directions.

Heat corn oil and sauté onion and garlic until soft. Add ½ cup cooked beans and mash them with the onion mixture until they are almost smooth. Add remaining beans and simmer about 30 minutes, or until thickened. Add salt, pepper, olive oil, and vinegar. Serve over hot rice and top with any or all of the suggested garnishes.

Serves 6

BROCCOLI AND CAULIFLOWER NEAPOLITAN

1 small cauliflower (about 1 pound)
1 small broccoli (about 1 pound)
1 tablespoon olive oil
2 cloves garlic, minced
1 teaspoon thyme
1 teaspoon basil
1 15-ounce can tomato puree
¼ teaspoon salt
½ teaspoon pepper
2 ounces parmesan cheese, freshly grated
2 ounces part-skim mozzarella cheese, grated
½ pound whole-wheat vermicelli (white may be substituted)
1 cup chopped fresh parsley

Wash cauliflower and broccoli and break into very small florets. Peel and slice broccoli stems with a paring knife.

Heat oil and sauté garlic, thyme, and basil for one minute. Add tomato puree, salt, pepper, and cauliflower and cook 5 minutes, covered, over medium-high heat. Add broccoli and cook for 20 minutes more over medium heat, uncovered. Remove from heat; add half the parmesan and half the mozzarella. Mix well.

Cook vermicelli while vegetable mixture is cooking. Drain vermicelli well and immediately spread onto a platter; pour cauliflower-broccoli mixture on top. Top with remaining parmesan and mozzarella. Sprinkle with parsley.

Serves 6

BROCCOLI-NOODLE CASSEROLE

2 cups chopped fresh broccoli
1 tablespoon margarine
2 tablespoons vegetable broth
1 pound fresh mushrooms, chopped
1 cup chopped onion
½ teaspoon salt
½ teaspoon pepper
¼ cup white wine
3 eggs, beaten
3 cups low-fat cottage cheese
1 cup low-fat yogurt
2 cloves garlic
1 teaspoon basil
8 ounces flat whole-wheat noodles (white may
    be substituted)
4 tablespoons bread crumbs
2 ounces grated cheddar cheese

Break broccoli into florets; peel and slice stems.

In a large skillet, melt margarine with broth and sauté broccoli, mushrooms, and onion for 10 minutes. Add salt, pepper, and wine. Stir to combine; remove from heat.

Beat eggs in a large bowl. Whisk in cottage cheese, yogurt, garlic, and basil. Cook noodles to al dente state. Drain noodles well and toss with cheese mixture. Add sautéed vegetables to cheese-noodle mixture.

Coat a 9″ × 13″ pan with cooking spray. Place broccoli-noodle mixture in pan; top with bread crumbs, and sprinkle with cheddar cheese.

Bake, covered, in a preheated 350°F oven for 30 minutes, then bake uncovered for 15 minutes more.

Serves 8

NUTRITIVE VALUES PER SERVING:

FAT	FIBER	VIT. A	VIT. C	CAL	CAL FROM FAT
8.92gm	9.09gm	1288 IU	39.4mg	324	25%

BROCCOLI QUICHE

1 pound broccoli, broken into florets, stems
  peeled and sliced
4 tablespoons unbleached white flour
2 eggs, beaten
2 ounces part-skim mozzarella, grated
¼ cup finely chopped parsley
½ teaspoon oregano
½ teaspoon basil
2 cups low-fat cottage cheese
1 tablespoon fresh lemon juice
½ teaspoon salt
¼ teaspoon pepper
⅓ cup seasoned italian bread crumbs

Steam broccoli until barely done; drain and chop coarsely.
Whisk flour with beaten eggs. Add broccoli and all remaining
ingredients except bread crumbs to eggs. Mix gently but thoroughly.
  Coat a rectangular pan (9″ × 13″ or smaller) with cooking
spray. Place broccoli mixture in pan; sprinkle top with bread
crumbs. Bake in a preheated 350°F oven for 35–40 minutes. Cool
2–3 minutes and cut into squares to serve.

Serves 4

NUTRITIVE VALUES PER SERVING:

FAT	FIBER	VIT. A	VIT. C	CAL	CAL FROM FAT
8.10gm	7.49gm	3450 IU	111mg	265	28%

BRUSSELS SPROUTS AND CHEESE BAKE

20 ounces brussels sprouts, fresh or frozen
2 cups low-fat cottage cheese
1 cup low-fat yogurt
$\frac{1}{2}$ cup sliced scallions
2 cloves garlic, minced
$\frac{1}{2}$ teaspoon paprika
$\frac{1}{2}$ teaspoon salt
$\frac{1}{4}$ teaspoon pepper
1 cup seasoned italian bread crumbs
2 ounces part-skim mozzarella, grated

Steam fresh sprouts until almost done. If using frozen sprouts, just defrost and drain them. Combine drained sprouts with all ingredients except bread crumbs and mozzarella. Mix well.

Place in a lightly oiled casserole dish; top with bread crumbs and sprinkle with mozzarella. Bake, uncovered, for 45 minutes in a preheated 300°F oven.

Serves 6

NUTRITIVE VALUES PER SERVING:

FAT	FIBER	VIT. A	VIT. C	CAL	CAL FROM FAT
4.71gm	3.05gm	736 IU	85.2mg	210	20%

CALIFORNIA BAKED BEANS

$1\frac{1}{2}$ tablespoons margarine or butter
2 cups chopped onion
1 cup chopped green bell pepper
2 teaspoons chili powder
1 teaspoon dijon mustard
$\frac{1}{2}$ teaspoon salt
$\frac{1}{2}$ teaspoon pepper
2 tablespoons brown sugar
6 ounces grated part-skim mozzarella cheese
2 cups chopped tomatoes
$\frac{1}{4}$ cup dry white wine
6 cups cooked pinto or kidney beans, drained

Heat margarine in a large pan. Sauté onion and green pepper in margarine for 5 minutes. Add chili powder, mustard, salt, pepper, and brown sugar. Off heat, add cheese, tomatoes, and wine to the sautéed onion mixture; stir in drained beans. Transfer to a large casserole coated with cooking spray. Cover and bake in a preheated 350°F oven for 45 minutes. Serve hot.

Serves 6

NUTRITIVE VALUES PER SERVING:

FAT	FIBER	VIT. A	VIT. C	CAL	CAL FROM FAT
8.55gm	20.4gm	420 IU	37.6mg	369	21%

CHEESE AND NOODLE PUDDING

8 ounces whole-wheat bow ties or other small-sized pasta (white may be substituted)
1½ cups low-fat milk
3 eggs, beaten
¾ cup chopped green bell pepper
¾ cup grated carrots
1¼ cups part-skim ricotta cheese
¾ cup sliced fresh mushrooms
¾ cup sliced scallions
3 cloves garlic, minced
¾ teaspoon basil
¼ teaspoon pepper
2 tablespoons freshly grated parmesan cheese

Cook pasta until tender; drain. Beat milk and eggs together. Add all remaining ingredients except parmesan, and mix well.

Pour into a lightly oiled 3-cup baking dish and sprinkle with parmesan cheese. Place in a larger pan filled with hot water to a 1 inch depth. Bake for 35 minutes in a preheated 350°F oven. Let set for a few minutes before serving.

Serves 6

NUTRITIVE VALUES PER SERVING:

FAT	FIBER	VIT. A	VIT. C	CAL	CAL FROM FAT
6.05gm	6.29gm	2674 IU	30.0mg	259	21%

CHEESE AND SPINACH WITH NOODLES

10 ounces whole-wheat flat noodles (white may
be substituted)
3 cups low-fat cottage cheese
½ cup chopped fresh parsley
2 scallions, sliced
½ teaspoon salt
¼ teaspoon pepper
1 teaspoon paprika
1 teaspoon oregano
1 tablespoon margarine or butter
2 tablespoons broth
1 cup chopped onion
2 cloves garlic, minced
3 tablespoons unbleached white flour
1½ cups vegetable broth
1 10-ounce package frozen chopped spinach,
defrosted and drained
4 ounces part-skim mozzarella cheese, grated

Cook noodles until tender; drain. Spread in a 9" × 13" pan coated
with cooking spray. Mix cottage cheese, parsley, scallions, salt,
pepper, paprika, and oregano. Spread cottage cheese mixture
over noodles.

Heat margarine with 2 tablespoons broth and sauté onions
and garlic for 5 minutes over medium heat. Add flour and cook
until blended, stirring constantly. Add 1½ cups broth and bring
to a boil; reduce heat and simmer 5 minutes, stirring constantly.
Add spinach; stir to combine. Spoon over noodles and cheese.
Top with mozzarella and bake in a preheated 350°F oven,
uncovered, for 20–25 minutes. Serve hot.

Serves 6

NUTRITIVE VALUES PER SERVING:

FAT	FIBER	VIT. A	VIT. C	CAL	CAL FROM FAT
8.20gm	9.30gm	4606 IU	23.0mg	397	19%

CHEESY SOYBEAN BAKE

1 tablespoon margarine or butter
2 tablespoons broth
1 cup chopped onion
3 cloves garlic, minced
½ pound fresh mushrooms, chopped
½ teaspoon basil
½ teaspoon thyme
½ teaspoon oregano
½ teaspoon salt
¼ teaspoon pepper
3 eggs, lightly beaten
2 cups low-fat cottage cheese
4 ounces grated part-skim mozzarella
2 cups cooked soybeans, drained (about 1 cup raw)
2 cups cooked brown rice (about ⅔ cup raw)
2 tablespoons soy sauce
2 medium tomatoes, thinly sliced
2 ounces freshly grated parmesan cheese
½ cup bread crumbs

Melt margarine with broth in a large pan; sauté onions, garlic, mushrooms, herbs, salt, and pepper for 5 minutes over medium heat. Combine eggs, cottage cheese, and mozzarella. Off heat, add sautéed vegetables to egg mixture. Add drained soybeans, rice, and soy sauce and spread mixture in a lightly oiled loaf pan. Top with sliced tomatoes, parmesan, and bread crumbs. Bake in a preheated 350°F oven for 40 minutes, uncovered. Let set a few minutes before serving.

Serves 8

NUTRITIVE VALUES PER SERVING:

FAT	FIBER	VIT. A	VIT. C	CAL	CAL FROM FAT
10.3gm	4.84gm	578 IU	10.1mg	289	32%

CHILI-CHEESE PIE

CRUST

2½ cups water
½ teaspoon salt
½ teaspoon chili powder
1⅓ cups cornmeal

FILLING

1 tablespoon corn or safflower oil
½ cup chopped onion
½ cup chopped green bell pepper
1 4-ounce can mild green chilies, drained
1 teaspoon oregano
½ teaspoon ground cumin
½ teaspoon chili powder
½ teaspoon salt
¼ teaspoon pepper
1½ cups cooked kidney beans, drained and
    chopped
½ cup corn, frozen or canned, drained
4 ounces grated part-skim mozzarella
2 ounces grated cheddar cheese
1 egg, beaten
¼ cup low-fat milk
2 medium tomatoes, thinly sliced

Combine water, salt, chili powder, and cornmeal in a saucepan and cook over medium heat until stiff (about 10 minutes), stirring frequently. Coat a 9" × 13" dish with cooking spray; line sides and bottom with cornmeal mixture.

Heat oil in a large skillet; sauté onion, green pepper, and chilies in the oil for 5 minutes over medium heat. Add oregano, cumin, chili powder, salt, and pepper. Remove from heat. Add beans and corn.

Combine the two cheeses. Mix egg and milk and add to the bean mixture with ⅓ of the cheese mixture. Spread ⅓ of the cheese mixture over bottom of crust. Spoon in bean filling and press down gently. Arrange sliced tomatoes over top and sprinkle with remaining cheese mixture. Bake, uncovered, for 35 minutes in a preheated 350°F oven. Cool for 5–10 minutes before cutting.

Serves 8

NUTRITIVE VALUES PER SERVING:

FAT	FIBER	VIT. A	VIT. C	CAL	CAL FROM FAT
7.78gm	5.92gm	753 IU	30.2mg	242	29%

COTTAGE CHEESE ENCHILADAS WITH GREEN SAUCE

3 cups low-fat cottage cheese
½ cup chopped fresh parsley
1½ teaspoons thyme
1½ teaspoons oregano
½ teaspoon salt
3 4-ounce cans diced mild green chilies, drained
1½ cups vegetable broth
10 large romaine lettuce leaves, torn into pieces
2 tablespoons corn or safflower oil
8 flour tortillas
4 ounces grated mozzarella cheese

Mix cottage cheese, parsley, thyme, oregano, and salt to make filling. To make sauce, process the chilies, broth, and lettuce in a blender until smooth. Heat oil in a skillet, add the sauce, and simmer 5 minutes.

Soften tortillas by heating on a griddle or frying pan. Fill tortillas with cottage cheese filling and roll up. Pour ½ of the sauce into a 9″ × 13″ pan and add the filled tortillas, seam side down. Cover with remaining sauce and sprinkle with mozzarella. Bake in a preheated 400°F oven for 20 minutes, uncovered.

Serves 8

Nutritive Values per Serving:

FAT	FIBER	VIT. A	VIT. C	CAL	CAL FROM FAT
9.46gm	1.88gm	992 IU	37.8mg	256	33%

CURRIED INDIAN-STYLE VEGETABLES

1 cup raw brown rice
1½ cups water
1 cup tomato puree
2 tablespoons oil
2 cups cubed unpeeled potatoes
1 cup sliced carrots
1 cup chopped tomatoes
1½ cups chopped onions
2 cups chopped cauliflower
½ teaspoon sugar
½ teaspoon salt
½ teaspoon curry powder
½ teaspoon ground cumin
½ teaspoon turmeric
½ teaspoon powdered ginger
¼ teaspoon pepper
¼ teaspoon cloves
1 16-ounce can garbanzo beans, drained
1 cup chopped green bell pepper
1 cup chopped unpeeled cucumber

Start rice, cooking according to package directions.

In a large pan, combine water, tomato puree, oil, potatoes, carrots, tomatoes, onions, cauliflower, sugar, salt, curry, cumin, turmeric, ginger, pepper, and cloves. Cook, covered, for 40 minutes over medium heat. Add garbanzo beans and simmer, uncovered, for 5 minutes to heat through. Serve over hot rice and pass chopped green pepper and cucumber as garnishes.

Serves 6

NUTRITIVE VALUES PER SERVING:

FAT	FIBER	VIT. A	VIT. C	CAL	CAL FROM FAT
7.74gm	12.1gm	3852 IU	87.4mg	357	20%

EGGPLANT PARMESAN

3 medium eggplants, peeled
1½ cups finely chopped onion
2 cloves garlic, minced
1 tablespoon olive oil
2 cups low-fat cottage cheese
3 ounces part-skim mozzarella, grated
½ cup bread crumbs
1 teaspoon oregano
1 teaspoon basil
1 teaspoon thyme
½ teaspoon salt
¼ teaspoon pepper
3 tomatoes, thinly sliced
2 cups Marinara Sauce (see Index)
1 ounce parmesan cheese, freshly grated

Preheat oven to 350°F. Slice eggplants and salt lightly. Place on a baking tray coated with cooking spray and bake 15 minutes or until tender.

Sauté onion and garlic in oil until soft. Remove pan from heat and add cottage cheese, mozzarella, bread crumbs, oregano, basil, thyme, salt, and pepper.

Coat a 9″ × 13″ pan with cooking spray; layer half of the eggplant slices in pan. Spread with cheese mixture. Top with other half of the eggplant slices. Place tomato slices on top of the eggplant. Pour Marinara Sauce over and sprinkle with parmesan. Bake for 25 minutes at 350°F, covered. Uncover and bake 10 minutes more. Let set a few minutes before serving.

Serves 8

Nutritive Values per Serving:

FAT	FIBER	VIT. A	VIT. C	CAL	CAL FROM FAT
6.27gm	4.56gm	571 IU	18.1mg	181	31%

LASAGNA PINWHEELS
WITH TWO SAUCES

16 ounces regular whole-wheat lasagna noodles
(not extra wide) (white may be substituted)
2 cups low-fat cottage cheese
1 cup part-skim ricotta cheese
1 ounce parmesan cheese, freshly grated
2 packages frozen chopped spinach, defrosted
and squeezed dry
½ teaspoon basil
1 teaspoon oregano
¼ teaspoon nutmeg
½ teaspoon salt
¼ teaspoon pepper
4 cups Marinara Sauce (see Index)
1¼ cups Light White Sauce (see Index), at room
temperature

Boil noodles for 10 minutes in a large pot. Drain carefully and
pat dry. Combine all remaining ingredients except sauces to
make filling. Spread filling along the length of each noodle and
roll up.

Place 2 cups Marinara Sauce on the bottom of a 9″ × 13″ pan.
Place noodles in pan on their ends (with one "curly" end up) and
spoon remaining Marinara Sauce over noodles. Bake in a preheated 350°F oven for 45 minutes. If pinwheels begin to brown,
lay a piece of foil loosely over them. Serve with about 2 tablespoons Light White Sauce spooned over each pinwheel.

Serves 10

Nutritive Values per Serving:

FAT	FIBER	VIT. A	VIT. C	CAL	CAL FROM FAT
7.38gm	8.75gm	6115 IU	22.1mg	360	18%

MANICOTTI

8 manicotti shells
1½ cups low-fat ricotta cheese
1 egg, beaten
1 10-ounce package frozen chopped spinach,
    defrosted and squeezed dry
¼ cup minced fresh parsley
3 tablespoons freshly grated parmesan cheese
½ teaspoon basil
½ teaspoon salt
½ teaspoon pepper
⅛ teaspoon nutmeg
¼ teaspoon garlic powder
4 cups Marinara Sauce (see Index)
3 tablespoons freshly grated parmesan cheese

Precook manicotti according to package directions for stuffing. Blend ricotta, egg, spinach, parsley, 3 tablespoons parmesan, basil, salt, pepper, nutmeg, and garlic powder until smooth. Stuff manicotti shells with the filling. Cover bottom of a 9″ × 13″ pan with 1 cup Marinara Sauce. Arrange shells on top of sauce in pan, in a single layer. Cover with remaining 3 cups sauce, combining any leftover filling with the sauce. Sprinkle with remaining parmesan, cover pan with foil, and bake in a pre-heated 375°F oven for 1 hour.

Makes 8 stuffed manicotti

NUTRITIVE VALUES PER SERVING:

FAT	FIBER	VIT. A	VIT. C	CAL	CAL FROM FAT
7.22gm	3.32gm	4377 IU	22.7mg	237	27%

MEATLESS CABBAGE ROLLS

1 head cabbage
1 tablespoon margarine
1 cup grated carrots
1 cup chopped onion
1½ cups cooked brown rice (about ½ cup raw)
½ teaspoon salt
¼ teaspoon pepper
¼ teaspoon cumin
¼ teaspoon celery seed
1 tablespoon fresh lemon juice
2 cups vegetable broth
6 ounces part-skim mozzarella cheese, grated
1 28-ounce can tomatoes, coarsely chopped,
  undrained

Remove core from cabbage, leaving head intact. Place cabbage head in a large kettle of boiling water. Cook, partly covered, for 10 minutes. Lift out carefully and drain. Remove 16–20 outer leaves, dry gently, and put aside.

To prepare filling, melt margarine and sauté carrots and onions for 5 minutes. Add rice, seasonings, and lemon juice and ½ cup of broth. Cover, and simmer for 15 minutes on low heat. Remove from heat, cool a bit, and add cheese.

Trim thick center rib from each reserved cabbage leaf to facilitate rolling. Place 3–4 tablespoons filling in center of each leaf and roll leaf up and around filling, tucking in sides. Rolls may be tied with thread or secured with toothpicks, if desired.

Place rolls, seam side down, in a 9″ × 13″ pan. Pour remaining broth and chopped tomatoes, with their juice, over the rolls. Cover and bake in a preheated 375°F oven for 1 hour. Uncover and bake 30 minutes more, basting frequently with juice.

For a thicker sauce, drain juice into a saucepan after cabbage rolls are done, and bring to a boil. Add 2 tablespoons cornstarch mixed with 2 tablespoons water and simmer until thickened. Serve hot.

Serves 8

NUTRITIVE VALUES PER SERVING:

FAT	FIBER	VIT. A	VIT. C	CAL	CAL FROM FAT
5.89gm	5.41gm	3216 IU	51.0mg	161	33%

MEXICAN RICE CRUST PIZZA

3 cups cooked brown rice (about 1 cup raw)
4 ounces part-skim mozzarella, grated
2 eggs, beaten
1 cup cooked kidney beans, chopped
1 13-ounce can Mexican tomatillos, drained, *or*
 1¼ cups red tomatoes, chopped and drained
⅓ cup finely chopped onion
2 cloves garlic, minced
1 4-ounce can diced mild green chilies, drained
⅓ cup chopped fresh cilantro (coriander)
½ teaspoon salt
1 teaspoon sugar
4 ounces monterey jack cheese, grated

TOPPINGS

½ cup green bell pepper slices
½ cup sliced mushrooms
½ cup sliced tomatoes
¼ cup sliced scallions

Combine rice, mozzarella, and eggs and spread in a 9″ × 13″ baking pan coated with cooking spray. Spread chopped beans over rice. To make sauce, chop tomatillos, onion, garlic, chilies, cilantro, salt, and sugar in a blender or food processor until smooth. Spread sauce over beans. Sprinkle with monterey jack cheese and the toppings. Bake in a preheated 375°F oven for 40 minutes. Cool for a few minutes and cut into squares.

Serves 8

NUTRITIVE VALUES PER SERVING:

FAT	FIBER	VIT. A	VIT. C	CAL	CAL FROM FAT
8.78gm	5.98gm	1054 IU	37.5mg	248	32%

PASTA PRIMAVERA

4 ounces whole-wheat pasta, small shells or bow
ties (white may be substituted)
1 cup chopped broccoli florets
1 cup peas, fresh or frozen, defrosted and
drained
1 cup thinly sliced red or green bell peppers
1 cup chopped tomatoes
2 scallions, sliced
½ cup chopped fresh parsley
¼ cup low-fat yogurt
2 tablespoons sour cream
2 tablespoons buttermilk
½ teaspoon salt
¼ teaspoon pepper
½ teaspoon oregano
½ teaspoon basil
4 ounces freshly grated parmesan cheese

Cook and drain pasta. Cool.

Cook broccoli and peas separately, just until crisp-tender.
Drain and cool. Combine pasta with broccoli, peas, peppers,
tomatoes, scallions, and parsley and toss gently but well.

Blend yogurt, sour cream, buttermilk, salt, pepper, oregano,
and basil together and add to pasta, tossing to coat. Add parmesan and toss gently to combine thoroughly. Refrigerate and
serve chilled.

Serves 4

NUTRITIVE VALUES PER SERVING:

FAT	FIBER	VIT. A	VIT. C	CAL	CAL FROM FAT
11.3gm	12.45gm	3053 IU	121mg	333	31%

PEPPER AND CHEESE BAKE

1½ cups bulgur (cracked wheat)
1½ cups chopped onions
1 tablespoon corn or safflower oil
1 tablespoon vegetable broth
4 cups chopped green bell peppers
1½ cups sliced mushrooms
1½ tablespoons sherry
1 teaspoon oregano
½ teaspoon salt
¼ teaspoon pepper
2 ounces crumbled feta cheese
1½ cups low-fat cottage cheese
4 eggs, beaten
Paprika

Soak bulgur in 1½ cups water for ½ hour; drain well. Sauté onions in oil and broth until translucent. Add peppers and mushrooms and cook until peppers are almost tender. Remove from heat. Add sherry, oregano, salt, and pepper to sautéed vegetables and mix well.

Combine feta with cottage cheese. Coat a 9" × 13" pan with cooking spray. Spread drained bulgur over bottom of pan and cover bulgur with vegetables, then with mixed cheeses. Pour beaten eggs over everything and sprinkle with paprika. Bake in a preheated 350°F oven for 40 minutes, uncovered. Let set for 10 minutes before cutting.

Serves 8

NUTRITIVE VALUES PER SERVING:

FAT	FIBER	VIT. A	VIT. C	CAL	CAL FROM FAT
7.66gm	5.21gm	564 IU	100mg	255	27%

POTATO-CABBAGE CASSEROLE

4 medium potatoes, unpeeled
1½ cups low-fat cottage cheese
¼ cup sour cream
¾ cup low-fat yogurt
1½ cups chopped onion
2 tablespoons margarine or butter
½ teaspoon marjoram
½ teaspoon salt
¼ teaspoon pepper
½ teaspoon paprika
4 cups chopped cabbage
2 tablespoons white wine

Cut potatoes into small cubes and steam until just tender. Drain and mash potatoes while still hot, adding cottage cheese, sour cream, and yogurt while mashing (use a potato masher or fork so potatoes don't get pulverized).

Sauté onions in margarine for 5 minutes. Add marjoram, salt, pepper, paprika, cabbage, and wine, stirring to combine well. Sauté until cabbage is tender, about 15 minutes. Add potato mixture and stir to combine. Spread into a casserole dish coated with cooking spray. Bake in a preheated 350°F oven for 40 minutes, covered, stirring halfway through.

Serves 6

NUTRITIVE VALUES PER SERVING:

FAT	FIBER	VIT. A	VIT. C	CAL	CAL FROM FAT
7.43gm	4.61gm	379 IU	42.1mg	221	30%

POTATO-CHEESE PANCAKES

These pancakes are delicious served with low-fat yogurt.

4 cups grated potatoes, unpeeled
6 ounces grated part-skim mozzarella cheese
.2 cups grated carrots
4 eggs, beaten
⅔ cup unbleached white flour
¼ cup minced onion
½ teaspoon salt
½ cup chopped fresh parsley
½ teaspoon pepper
2 tablespoons fresh lemon juice
2 cloves garlic, minced

Lightly salt grated potatoes and let drain 15 minutes. Squeeze potatoes to get rid of excess water. Combine drained potatoes with remaining ingredients to make batter.

Heat a nonstick pan, or one coated with cooking spray, to medium-high. Use approximately ¼ cup batter for each pancake, pressing down to make pancake thin. Fry about 2 minutes on each side until browned and crisp on both sides. Keep cooked pancakes warm while frying the remainder by placing them in a single layer on a baking sheet in a warming oven.

Serves 8

NUTRITIVE VALUES PER SERVING:

FAT	FIBER	VIT. A	VIT. C	CAL	CAL FROM FAT
6.47gm	4.39gm	4647 IU	21.9mg	198	30%

SOUTH AMERICAN PEPPERS AND CHEESE

6 medium bell peppers (red, green, or a combination)
1½ tablespoons olive oil
1½ cups thinly sliced onions
3 medium cloves garlic, minced
½ teaspoon salt
1 teaspoon ground cumin
1 teaspoon ground coriander
4 ounces part-skim mozzarella cheese, grated
2 eggs
1 cup low-fat yogurt
⅓ cup sour cream
Paprika
1½ cups raw brown rice

Slice peppers into strips. Heat oil in a heavy pan. Sauté onions and garlic with salt, cumin, and coriander. When onions are soft, add pepper strips. Sauté over low heat for 10 minutes.

Coat a deep casserole dish with cooking spray. Spread half the bell pepper mixture in the dish; top with half the mozzarella. Repeat layers. Mix eggs, yogurt, and sour cream and pour over mixture in casserole. Sprinkle with paprika.

Start rice, cooking according to package directions. Bake casserole, covered, for 30 minutes in a preheated 375°F oven. Uncover and bake 15 minutes more. Serve with hot rice.

Serves 6

NUTRITIVE VALUES PER SERVING:

FAT	FIBER	VIT. A	VIT. C	CAL	CAL FROM FAT
12.8gm	5.28gm	805 IU	149mg	357	32%

SOUTH AMERICAN SQUASH

4 cups butternut (or hubbard or banana)
   squash, cut into small cubes
1 tablespoon corn or safflower oil
1 cup chopped onion
2 large cloves garlic, minced
¾ teaspoon chili powder
¾ teaspoon ground coriander
⅛ teaspoon cayenne pepper
½ teaspoon salt
⅛ teaspoon pepper
2 cups corn (drained if canned or frozen)
2 eggs, beaten
2 ounces mozzarella cheese, grated
1½ ounces cheddar cheese, grated

Steam cubed squash until done. In oil, sauté onions and garlic with chili powder, coriander, cayenne, salt, and pepper until onions are translucent. Cover and cook for 5 minutes over low heat. Off heat, add cubed squash, corn, eggs, and mozzarella to onion mixture. Toss gently until well blended. Spread in a 2-quart dish coated with cooking spray; top with cheddar cheese.

Bake in a preheated 350°F oven for 20 minutes covered, then 20 minutes uncovered.

Serves 6

NUTRITIVE VALUES PER SERVING:

FAT	FIBER	VIT. A	VIT. C	CAL	CAL FROM FAT
8.89gm	9.56gm	6162 IU	23.5mg	238	34%

SPAGHETTI SQUASH AND RICE QUICHE

2 cups cooked spaghetti squash
1 cup low-fat cottage cheese
2 eggs
½ cup low-fat milk
½ teaspoon salt
¼ teaspoon pepper
2 cups cooked brown rice (about ⅔ cup raw)
2 ounces grated part-skim mozzarella
1 cup tomato sauce or Marinara Sauce (see Index)

To cook spaghetti squash, cut lengthwise, remove seeds, pierce skin with a fork, and bake, cut side down, at 350°F for 45 minutes. In blender or food processor, combine cottage cheese and eggs; blend until smooth. Add squash, milk, salt, and pepper and blend until smooth.

Pat rice on bottom of a 10″ round × 2″ baking dish coated with cooking spray. Pour squash mixture over rice; sprinkle with cheese. Bake at 350°F for 45 minutes, or until set. Let set for a few minutes before cutting and serving. Serve with tomato sauce or Marinara Sauce.

Serves 4

NUTRITIVE VALUES PER SERVING:

FAT	FIBER	VIT. A	VIT. C	CAL	CAL FROM FAT
7.85gm	5.60gm	1390 IU	21.7mg	291	24%

SPAGHETTI WITH SPINACH AND MUSHROOMS

1 package frozen chopped spinach
½ pound fresh mushrooms
1 tablespoon fresh lemon juice
1 tablespoon margarine or butter
2 cloves garlic, minced
2 tablespoons madeira wine
1 cup low-fat milk
½ teaspoon salt
¼ teaspoon pepper
½ pound whole-wheat spaghetti (white may be substituted)
2 ounces freshly grated parmesan cheese

Defrost spinach and drain well (save juice for other uses). Wash mushrooms, trim ends, and slice thinly. Add lemon juice to mushrooms and mix well.

Melt margarine in a large skillet; add garlic and madeira and cook for 3 minutes. Add mushrooms and cook 5 minutes more, then add milk, salt, and pepper and bring to a boil. Add spinach, stir to combine all ingredients well, and simmer for 5 minutes. Remove from heat; keep warm while cooking spaghetti.

Cook spaghetti al dente and drain. Immediately combine spinach and mushroom mixture with spaghetti and toss to combine well. Top each serving with ¼ of the parmesan cheese.

Serves 4

NUTRITIVE VALUES PER SERVING:

FAT	FIBER	VIT. A	VIT. C	CAL	CAL FROM FAT
9.76gm	14.59gm	6659 IU	26.0mg	390	23%

SPINACH-CHEESE DUMPLINGS

2 tablespoons margarine or butter

1 10-ounce package frozen chopped spinach, defrosted and drained well

½ cup part-skim ricotta cheese

½ teaspoon salt

⅛ teaspoon pepper

¼ teaspoon nutmeg

2 eggs, beaten

½ cup unbleached white flour

¼ cup freshly grated parmesan cheese

1 teaspoon basil

¼ teaspoon sugar

1 clove garlic, minced

6 ounces whole-wheat noodles (white may be substituted)

3 cups Marinara Sauce (see Index)

Heat margarine; add spinach and sauté over medium-low heat until moisture has evaporated. Turn heat to low, stir in ricotta, salt, pepper, and nutmeg; cook 5 more minutes, stirring. Remove from heat and cool a bit.

Mix in eggs, flour, parmesan, basil, sugar, and garlic and blend very well. Refrigerate for 1–2 hours.

To make dumplings, boil 4 quarts water in a big pot. With 2 spoons, shape chilled dumpling mixture into 24 balls and drop in boiling water (add slowly, so water remains boiling). Boil for 10 minutes. Lift out with a slotted spoon and drain carefully. Cook noodles while boiling dumplings. Heat Marinara Sauce at the same time. Serve dumplings and drained, hot noodles with Marinara Sauce spooned over both.

Serves 6

NUTRITIVE VALUES PER SERVING:

FAT	FIBER	VIT. A	VIT. C	CAL	CAL FROM FAT
10.3gm	7.33gm	5339 IU	25.8mg	318	29%

SPINACH-CHEESE PANCAKES

PANCAKE BATTER

2 eggs, beaten

1 tablespoon margarine or butter, melted and
   cooled

1¾ cups low-fat milk

2 packages frozen chopped spinach, defrosted
   and squeezed dry

6 ounces part-skim mozzarella, grated

½ cup sliced scallions

½ teaspoon salt

¼ teaspoon sugar

¼ teaspoon pepper

¼ teaspoon oregano

1 cup unbleached white flour

OREGANO-YOGURT SAUCE

1 cup low-fat yogurt

½ teaspoon oregano

¼ teaspoon salt

¼ teaspoon pepper

2 tablespoons minced scallions

To make pancake batter, combine eggs, margarine, and milk.
Add spinach to milk mixture and combine thoroughly. Add
cheese, scallions, and seasonings and mix. Add flour and mix
until well blended.

Using approximately 2 tablespoons batter for each pancake,
fry on a skillet or griddle coated with cooking spray until golden
and crispy on both sides. Combine all ingredients for Oregano
Yogurt Sauce and mix well. Serve with pancakes.

Serves 4

NUTRITIVE VALUES PER SERVING:

FAT	FIBER	VIT. A	VIT. C	CAL	CAL FROM FAT
9.32gm	11.2gm	13,446 IU	49.7mg	309	27%

VEGETARIAN CHILI CASSEROLE

1 cup raw brown rice
2 cups water
1 15-ounce can tomato sauce
1 15-ounce can tomatoes with juice, undrained,
    broken with fork
1 cup chopped onion
½ cup chopped green bell pepper
½ cup chopped fresh parsley
1 teaspoon oregano
½ teaspoon ground cumin
½ teaspoon ground coriander
2 large cloves garlic, minced
¼ teaspoon pepper
1 tablespoon chili powder
2 16-ounce cans kidney beans, drained
8 ounces grated part-skim mozzarella cheese

Mix together all ingredients except cheese in a large saucepan.
Bring to a boil; cover and cook over medium-low heat until rice
is tender, about 1 hour, stirring occasionally. Sprinkle with
cheese, and serve immediately.

Serves 8

NUTRITIVE VALUES PER SERVING:

FAT	FIBER	VIT. A	VIT. C	CAL	CAL FROM FAT
5.70gm	7.41gm	1579 IU	38.9mg	244	21%

VEGETARIAN LASAGNA

1 cup part-skim ricotta cheese
1 cup low-fat cottage cheese
½ cup finely chopped fresh parsley
2 cloves garlic, minced
¼ teaspoon nutmeg
½ teaspoon pepper
4 cups Marinara Sauce (see Index)
12 whole-wheat lasagna noodles, cooked al
    dente and drained (white may be
    substituted)
½ pound grated low-fat mozzarella
¼ cup freshly grated parmesan cheese

Mix ricotta, cottage cheese, parsley, garlic, nutmeg, and pepper to make filling. Spread 1 cup Marinara Sauce over bottom of a 9″ × 13″ pan. Lay 4 lasagna noodles over the sauce. Put small mounds of the filling over noodles, about every 2 inches, using about ½ of the mixture. Cover with 1 cup of the sauce. Sprinkle half of the mozzarella cheese over the sauce.

Top first layer with 4 more noodles; cover with remaining filling and 1 cup more sauce. Sprinkle with remaining mozzarella. Put last 4 noodles on top. Cover with last cup of sauce and sprinkle with parmesan cheese. Bake in a preheated 375°F oven for 45 minutes, uncovering during the last 10 minutes. Let stand 5–10 minutes before dishing up.

Serves 8

NUTRITIVE VALUES PER SERVING:

FAT	FIBER	VIT. A	VIT. C	CAL	CAL FROM FAT
10.3gm	1.72gm	1814 IU	19.1mg	363	26%

6
Vegetables

Acorn Squash in the Shell
Apple-Cranberry Acorn Squash
Baked Squash
Bean Cakes
Bourbon-Orange Sweet Potatoes
Braised Fresh Tomatoes
Brussels Sprouts and Chestnuts
Cabbage with Noodles
Carrots and Cabbage, Mandarin Style
Carrots in Garlic Sauce
Creamed Cabbage
Creamed Spinach Bake
Curried Lentils
Garlic Sautéed Spinach
Herbed Beans
Honey-Baked Rutabaga
Italian Vegetable Stew
Julienne of Turnips and Carrots
Lemon Broccoli
Marinated Carrots
Mustard Cream Broccoli and Carrots

Onions Filled with Spinach
Oven French Fries
Ratatouille
Romanian Vegetable Casserole
Scalloped Potatoes and Carrots
Southern Greens and Turnips
Specially Seasoned Tomatoes
Spinach-Filled Tomatoes
Spinach Pancakes
Stir-Fried Broccoli
Stuffed White Potatoes
Sweet and Tart Lentils
Sweet Potato and Carrot Mold
Sweet Potato Fries
Sweet Potato Pancakes
Sweet Potato-Rice Bake
Sweet Potatoes with Apples
Swiss Chard Fritters
Walnut-Stuffed Sweet Potatoes
White Beans
Winter Vegetable Medley

Vegetables

Nature's bounty provides an eye-catching array of colorful vegetables—fresh leafy spinach, sweet baby carrots, bright broccoli florets, luscious beefsteak tomatoes—that gratify our senses and keep us healthy. Plain or fancy, steamed, sautéed, stir-fried, or baked, they rank among the best foods on a cancer risk–reduction eating plan.

Fruits and vegetables play an extremely important role in protecting the body from certain cancers. The most significant of the vegetables are those high in beta-carotene (which converts to vitamin A in the body), vitamin C, and indoles. Vegetables high in beta-carotene (or vitamin A) come in two colors: yellow-orange and dark green. Vegetables with the darkest colors tend to contain the most beta-carotene. Carrots, sweet potatoes, pumpkin, winter squash, and red peppers stand out in the yellow-orange group; swiss chard, spinach, broccoli, kale, and turnip greens top members of the dark green group.

Broccoli, cabbage, brussels sprouts, green peppers, potatoes, and most dark green leafy vegetables all contain good amounts of vitamin C. Indoles are contained in cruciferous vegetables, which include cabbage, kale, brussels sprouts, turnips, mustard and turnip greens, and cauliflower. Notice that several of the cruciferous vegetables are also listed as good sources of vitamins A and C.

This chapter shows you many ways to prepare these wonderfully healthful vegetables. We use fresh vegetables in most of the recipes—they are certainly tastier and more attractive than packaged ones. But sometimes the frozen variety is all that is available. Frozen vegetables do have this advantage: they can be stored for months and used when needed, and current methods of quick freezing usually ensure maximum vitamin content.

For the sake of keeping fat intake per meal to no more than 30%, use the simple rule of *plain entrée/fancy vegetable*. Applying this rule gives you leeway with salad dressings and side dishes. If you are planning a low-fat entrée such as poached chicken or broiled fish, you have room to enjoy some of our creamy vegetable dishes, or those made with a little more oil or margarine. Even these vegetable dishes are low in fat (if you maintain portion size!).

Begin with some of the simplest vegetable dishes: Garlic-Sautéed Spinach is quick, easy, and among the most flavorful recipes in the book. Fresh spinach, fresh garlic (even if you think you don't like it), a little broth, margarine, salt, and pepper—and it's ready.

The cabbage dishes are also simple and answer the question: What do you do with cabbage except serve it with corned beef on St. Patrick's Day? Both Cabbage with Noodles and Creamed Cabbage are easy to prepare and will agreeably surprise those of you who never cook this tasty vegetable.

To follow the *plain entrée/fancy vegetable* rule, prepare Italian Vegetable Stew, Mustard Cream Broccoli and Carrots, Ratatouille, or Creamed Spinach Bake to accompany a piece of poached chicken or fish or a slice of lean meat. Or use some of our "company" dishes: Lemon Broccoli, Specially Seasoned Tomatoes, Julienne of Turnips and Carrots, Onions Filled with Spinach, or Walnut-Stuffed Sweet Potatoes.

Potato lovers, rejoice! Both white and sweet potatoes rank high on a cancer risk–reduction eating plan. White potatoes contain vitamin C and are a good source of fiber. Sweet potatoes are extremely high in beta-carotene—one potato will supply you with almost two times the recommended daily allowance of vitamin A—and also contains dietary fiber along with many other essential nutrients. Eat the skins of new potatoes and well-scrubbed baking potatoes—they also contain fiber and vitamins. Before you bake potatoes, remove black marks and buds, and pierce several times with a fork to allow steam to release while baking.

In this chapter are some low-fat variations on high-fat white-potato favorites: Oven French Fries, Stuffed White Potatoes, Scalloped Potatoes and Carrots.

Don't save sweet potatoes just for Thanksgiving dinner—serve them often in casseroles such as Sweet Potato–Rice Bake, or Bourbon-Orange Sweet Potatoes. Try Sweet Potato Fries as an interesting alternative to Oven French Fries. You can also bake sweet potatoes as you would regular white potatoes. Instead of drowning them in butter, scoop out the insides after they are done, add a teaspoon of margarine and a tablespoon of low-fat ricotta cheese, mash, restuff the potato shell, and bake for a few more minutes. They taste creamy and sweet, and go well with chicken or veal.

Generally, yams have a deeper orange color and taste a little sweeter than sweet potatoes. Depending on availability, you can use these vegetables interchangeably—it is only a matter of personal taste. (You may find yams more appealing in casserole dishes because of their bright color.)

We hope to have tempted your palate with some new and interesting vegetable dishes.

Now, the best ways to prepare vegetables:

COOKING METHODS
Peeling and Seeding Tomatoes

To peel and seed fresh tomatoes, immerse them in boiling water for one to two minutes. Immediately plunge into cold water, then peel skins off tomatoes—they will literally fall away from the sides. Cut skinned tomatoes in half horizontally: squeeze out seeds and discard. The tomatoes are now ready to chop.

Steaming

Invest in a collapsible metal steamer if you don't already have one. They are inexpensive, easy to store, and ensure a foolproof method to cook most vegetables to perfection. Steaming also locks in vitamins. To steam vegetables, place steamer in a large pan with about an inch of water; bring water to a boil. Place vegetables in steamer basket and cover pan with a tightly fitting lid. Reduce heat to medium; water should stay lightly boiling. Don't lift the lid until vegetables are done.

Cooking time depends on the size and thickness of the vegetables. Leafy greens, such as spinach, kale, swiss chard, and turnip greens should cook 1–2 minutes if the leaves are left whole. Cabbage quarters, whole carrots (unpeeled and scrubbed), brussels sprouts, broccoli with stalks, and large chunks of squash take 15–25 minutes, depending on size. Rutabagas (cut into large chunks), whole new potatoes, and whole cauliflower cook in 20–30 minutes. Serve steamed vegetables with just a sprinkling of fresh lemon juice or chopped parsley to accompany a rich entrée.

Stir-Frying

Stir-fried vegetables retain almost all of their vitamin content, and remain crisp yet tender cooked by this method. To stir-fry, heat a wok or large metal pan on high. When the metal is hot enough to make a drop of water sizzle, coat the wok or pan with a minimal amount of corn or peanut oil—both are good for high-heat cooking. (Don't use olive oil; it will smoke and burn.) Add vegetables and cook on high until done. Cooking time will be a matter of minutes. The curved sides of the wok make it easy to rotate vegetables so they will cook evenly.

For a quick Chinese dish, you can make a glaze with water and cornstarch (see Stir-Fried Broccoli). You can also turn stir-fried vegetables into a meal by adding small strips of lean beef, pieces of poultry or fish, or cubed tofu flavored with soy sauce. Almost all vegetables can be stir-fried (tomatoes are the exception—they just wilt when heated). Steam thick or dense vegetables like turnips and cauliflower first to minimize cooking time needed in the wok. When stir-frying combinations, cook the thicker vegetables first, adding the thinner, faster-cooking ones last. Simple stir-fried vegetables are appropriate with any entrée, plain or fancy.

A Few Don'ts:

- Don't cook vegetables in an excessive amount of water—they lose vitamins and become soggy.
- Don't overcook vegetables either by boiling, baking, or steaming—they lose flavor, texture, and some vitamins.
- Don't overseason; you want to taste the vegetable, not the spices.

ACORN SQUASH IN THE SHELL

3 small acorn squash
1 teaspoon fresh lemon juice
¼ teaspoon allspice
½ teaspoon cinnamon
1 tablespoon margarine or butter
2 tablespoons brown sugar
2 tablespoons sherry

Cut squash in half lengthwise and scoop out seeds. Place cut side down on baking pan and pour ½ inch of water in pan. Bake in a preheated 375°F oven for 30 minutes. Remove from oven and scoop out pulp, leaving enough pulp for shell to hold its shape. Mix pulp with remaining ingredients and fill shells. Place on baking pan. Cover with foil and bake in a 375°F oven for 25 minutes. Serve hot.

Serves 6

NUTRITIVE VALUES PER SERVING:

FAT	FIBER	VIT. A	VIT. C	CAL	CAL FROM FAT
2.10gm	5.80gm	898 IU	21.3mg	69.2	27%

APPLE-CRANBERRY ACORN SQUASH

4 small acorn squash
2 medium unpeeled apples, chopped
½ cup fresh cranberries
¼ cup brown sugar
1 tablespoon Grand Marnier or orange juice
1 tablespoon melted margarine or butter
2 tablespoons chopped almonds

Cut squash in half, lengthwise. Remove seeds and place squash in a baking dish, cut side down. Pour ½ inch of water into dish. Bake in a preheated 375°F oven for 40 minutes.

Mix remaining ingredients together in a bowl for the filling. Turn squash cavity-side up and stuff with filling mixture. Bake for 30 more minutes, or until tender.

Serves 8

NUTRITIVE VALUES PER SERVING:

FAT	FIBER	VIT. A	VIT. C	CAL	CAL FROM FAT
2.63gm	4.72gm	490 IU	13.2mg	88.9	27%

BAKED SQUASH

1 3-pound pumpkin or other winter squash
2 tablespoons margarine or butter, melted
2 tablespoons vegetable or chicken broth
½ teaspoon salt
½ teaspoon pepper
1 cup finely chopped parsley

Cut pumpkin into 8 pieces and bake on a cookie sheet in a preheated 350°F oven for 45 minutes. Remove pumpkin meat from rind and cut into cubes. Toss with margarine, broth, salt, pepper, and parsley. Serve hot.

Serves 8

NUTRITIVE VALUES PER SERVING:

FAT	FIBER	VIT. A	VIT. C	CAL	CAL FROM FAT
3.60gm	8.23gm	7900 IU	35.2mg	136	24%

BEAN CAKES

Bean Cakes are a good alternative to ordinary refried beans.
Top with low-fat yogurt and salsa for an easy snack or lunch.

3 cups cooked pinto or kidney beans, drained
well
¼ teaspoon cayenne pepper
2 cloves garlic, minced
½ teaspoon salt
2 tablespoons margarine or butter

Chop beans coarsely and add cayenne, garlic, and salt. Mix until well combined. With hands, form into 8 flat cakes and sauté in margarine for 5 minutes on each side, or until golden brown.

Serves 8

NUTRITIVE VALUES PER SERVING:

FAT	FIBER	VIT. A	VIT. C	CAL	CAL FROM FAT
3.23gm	7.05gm	121 IU	0mg	119	24%

BOURBON-ORANGE SWEET POTATOES

4 pounds sweet potatoes
2 tablespoons margarine or butter
⅓ cup low-fat milk
¼ cup bourbon
¼ cup orange juice
¼ cup brown sugar
½ teaspoon salt
½ teaspoon pumpkin pie spice
¼ cup chopped pecans

Cook, cool, peel, and mash sweet potatoes. Add all remaining ingredients except pecans and beat until fluffy. Coat baking dish with cooking spray and spoon potato mixture into dish. Sprinkle with pecans and bake in a preheated 350°F oven for 40 minutes.

This may be made a day or two ahead and refrigerated. Increase baking time to 50 minutes for chilled potatoes.

Serves 8

NUTRITIVE VALUES PER SERVING:

FAT	FIBER	VIT. A	VIT. C	CAL	CAL FROM FAT
6.82gm	6.28gm	18,092 IU	43mg	358	17%

BRAISED FRESH TOMATOES

A variation of a classic French garnish, these flavorful tomatoes can be used as a vegetable, or as an accompaniment to egg dishes, other vegetables, plain chicken, or fish.

½ cup sliced scallions
1⅓ cups chopped onions
1 tablespoon margarine or butter
3 pounds ripe tomatoes, peeled, seeded, and
   diced (to peel and seed, see page 224)
6 cloves garlic, minced
3 bay leaves
¼ teaspoon thyme
½ teaspoon salt
¼ teaspoon pepper

Sauté scallions and onions in margarine until transparent. Add remaining ingredients and simmer, covered, for 1 hour. May be served chilled, at room temperature, or heated.

These tomatoes will keep in the refrigerator, covered, for a few days.

Serves 8

NUTRITIVE VALUES PER SERVING:

FAT	FIBER	VIT. A	VIT. C	CAL	CAL FROM FAT
1.72gm	3.11gm	1594 IU	40.1mg	55.1	28%

BRUSSELS SPROUTS AND CHESTNUTS

2 pounds fresh brussels sprouts
8 ounces fresh chestnuts
4 teaspoons margarine or butter
2 tablespoons vegetable or chicken broth
½ teaspoon salt
¼ teaspoon pepper

Cut an X in the root of each sprout and steam until tender (don't overcook). Cut a thin strip off the shell of each chestnut. Bring a pot of water to boiling, add chestnuts, and simmer for 15 minutes. Plunge chestnuts into cold water, then remove skins (large chestnuts may be cut in half). Heat margarine with broth and gently sauté sprouts and chestnuts together until heated through. Add salt and pepper and serve.

Serves 8

NUTRITIVE VALUES PER SERVING:

FAT	FIBER	VIT. A	VIT. C	CAL	CAL FROM FAT
3.13gm	5.19gm	602 IU	100mg	103	27%

CABBAGE WITH NOODLES

2 cups flat whole-wheat noodles (about 6 ounces)
½ tablespoon olive oil
1 tablespoon margarine or butter
1 tablespoon vegetable or chicken broth
¾ cup grated carrots
½ cup chopped red onion
2 cups grated cabbage
½ teaspoon salt
¼ teaspoon celery seed
¼ teaspoon garlic powder
¼ teaspoon pepper
½ cup chopped fresh parsley

Start noodles, cooking according to package directions. Drain well and toss with olive oil. Keep warm until vegetables are ready.

While noodles are cooking, melt margarine with broth in a large skillet and sauté carrots, onion, and cabbage on medium heat for 5 minutes. Add cooked noodles, seasonings, and parsley and gently toss. Serve immediately.

Serves 6

NUTRITIVE VALUES PER SERVING:

FAT	FIBER	VIT. A	VIT. C	CAL	CAL FROM FAT
3.65gm	5.44gm	2580 IU	22.5mg	158	21%

CARROTS AND CABBAGE, MANDARIN STYLE

2 tablespoons vegetable or chicken broth
⅔ cup chopped scallions
1 cup grated carrots
¼ pound fresh mushrooms, sliced
2 large cloves garlic, minced
2 tablespoons fresh minced ginger
6 cups grated cabbage
1½ teaspoons Chinese sesame oil (found in
    Oriental section of market)
1 tablespoon soy sauce

Heat broth in a large nonstick pan and cook scallions, carrots, mushrooms, garlic, and ginger for 2 minutes. Add cabbage and stir to coat cabbage with the scallion mixture. Add sesame oil and soy sauce and stir to coat thoroughly. Reduce heat to low, cover, and cook 5 minutes.

Serves 6

NUTRITIVE VALUES PER SERVING:

FAT	FIBER	VIT. A	VIT. C	CAL	CAL FROM FAT
1.44gm	4.75gm	3043 IU	40.1mg	41.7	31%

CARROTS IN GARLIC SAUCE

1 pound carrots, sliced
3 cloves garlic, quartered
1 teaspoon margarine or butter, well chilled
¼ cup vegetable or chicken broth
½ cup parsley

Steam carrots about 5 minutes, until just done. Drain and arrange in a shallow baking dish. Bury garlic quarters in among carrot slices, taking care to distribute them evenly. Dot with margarine, cut into several pieces, and pour broth over. Bake in preheated 350°F oven for 20 minutes, or until tender. Remove garlic and stir. Toss with parsley and serve.

Serves 6

NUTRITIVE VALUES PER SERVING:

FAT	FIBER	VIT. A	VIT. C	CAL	CAL FROM FAT
.81gm	3.77gm	8391 IU	12.9mg	26.3	28%

CREAMED CABBAGE

1 head green cabbage (about 1½ pounds), grated
1 teaspoon margarine
1 tablespoon unbleached white flour
1 teaspoon thyme
5 teaspoons vegetable broth
⅔ cup low-fat milk
½ teaspoon dijon mustard
½ teaspoon salt
¼ teaspoon pepper

Steam cabbage until just tender. Drain very well. Heat margarine in a large frying pan and stir in flour and thyme. Cook until blended, using a fork or whisk. Slowly add broth and milk and boil, whisking long enough to thicken slightly. Add mustard and stir to combine, then stir in cabbage and toss to coat well. Cook only until cabbage is tender. Season with salt and pepper.

Serves 4

NUTRITIVE VALUES PER SERVING:

FAT	FIBER	VIT. A	VIT. C	CAL	CAL FROM FAT
2.12gm	5.23gm	374 IU	81.6mg	76.3	25%

CREAMED SPINACH BAKE

1 10-ounce package frozen chopped spinach
1 whole egg, beaten
2 teaspoons margarine or butter
1 tablespoon broth
½ cup chopped scallions
½ cup chopped mushrooms
½ cup grated carrots
2 tablespoons unbleached white flour
¾ cup evaporated skim milk
½ teaspoon salt
¼ teaspoon pepper
⅛ teaspoon nutmeg

Defrost spinach and squeeze dry (save juice for soup). Using a fork, mix spinach thoroughly with beaten egg. Melt margarine with broth in a skillet and add scallions; sauté until softened but not browned. Add mushrooms and carrots and cook about 5 minutes over low heat or until liquid is evaporated. Add flour and stir to coat vegetables. Add evaporated milk and bring to a boil, stirring. Reduce heat and stir 2–3 minutes until mixture is thickened.

Remove from heat and stir in egg-spinach mixture. Season with salt, pepper, and nutmeg. Transfer to a standard-sized loaf pan coated with cooking spray. Bake in a preheated 350°F oven for 25 minutes, or until firm. Cut into squares and serve.

Serves 4

NUTRITIVE VALUES PER SERVING:

FAT	FIBER	VIT. A	VIT. C	CAL	CAL FROM FAT
3.75gm	6.34gm	8777 IU	20.8mg	118	29%

CURRIED LENTILS

Curried lentils are traditionally served with dishes of chopped cucumber, chopped onion, chopped tomato, and chutney on the side.

1 cup dried lentils
1 tablespoon margarine
1 tablespoon broth
½ cup chopped onion
½ cup grated carrots
1 tablespoon curry powder
1 tablespoon unbleached white flour
¼ cup water
1½ cups chicken broth
½ teaspoon pepper
¼ teaspoon sugar

GARNISHES

Chopped cucumber
Chopped onion
Chopped tomato
Chutney

Simmer lentils in enough water to cover for 30 minutes; don't overcook. Drain lentils well and set aside. Melt margarine with broth in a skillet. Add onion and carrots and stir until soft. Sprinkle with curry powder and flour and stir to combine. Add ¼ cup water and simmer for 10 minutes, covered. Add lentils, broth, pepper, and sugar and heat over low heat for 10 more minutes; add a bit more broth if needed. May be served over rice, accompanied by dishes of garnishes.

Serves 6

NUTRITIVE VALUES PER SERVING:

FAT	FIBER	VIT. A	VIT. C	CAL	CAL FROM FAT
2.58gm	4.54gm	1469 IU	4.36mg	137	17%

GARLIC SAUTEED SPINACH

2 teaspoons margarine
1 tablespoon vegetable or chicken broth
2 cloves garlic, minced
2 pounds fresh spinach, washed and well dried
½ teaspoon salt
¼ teaspoon pepper

Melt margarine with broth over medium heat and add garlic. Cook 2 minutes. Add spinach and sauté over high heat just until limp. Season with salt and pepper and serve immediately.

Serves 4

NUTRITIVE VALUES PER SERVING:

FAT	FIBER	VIT. A	VIT. C	CAL	CAL FROM FAT
2.64gm	16.0gm	18,470 IU	115mg	75.9	31%

HERBED BEANS

1 tablespoon olive oil
1 tablespoon margarine
2 tablespoons fresh lemon juice
½ cup chopped scallions
½ teaspoon oregano
½ teaspoon thyme
½ teaspoon salt
3 cups cooked kidney, pinto, or navy beans, well
drained (1 cup raw)

Heat oil and margarine; add lemon juice, scallions, and seasonings and simmer for 10 minutes. Add beans and simmer, gently,
10 minutes more. Serve hot.
  Leftover beans may be chilled and served as a bean salad.

Serves 6

NUTRITIVE VALUES PER SERVING:

FAT	FIBER	VIT. A	VIT. C	CAL	CAL FROM FAT
4.65gm	9.97gm	.251 IU	5.00mg	154	27%

HONEY-BAKED RUTABAGA

1 tablespoon margarine
½ cup white wine
2 tablespoons honey
1 tablespoon brown sugar
1 large rutabaga (or 2 large turnips), cubed

Melt margarine; add wine, honey, and brown sugar. Place cubed
rutabaga in a casserole and cover with honey-margarine mixture. Bake in a preheated 325°F oven for 1 hour tightly covered,
or until tender.

Serves 4

NUTRITIVE VALUES PER SERVING:

FAT	FIBER	VIT. A	VIT. C	CAL	CAL FROM FAT
3.00gm	3.6gm	822 IU	27.0mg	135	20%

ITALIAN VEGETABLE STEW

3 unpeeled medium potatoes, cubed
1 medium onion, coarsely chopped
3 small zucchini, sliced
1 green pepper, seeded and cubed
1 tablespoon olive oil
⅓ cup broth
2 cloves garlic, minced
½ teaspoon oregano
½ teaspoon basil
½ teaspoon salt
¼ teaspoon pepper

Place all ingredients into a heavy saucepan. Cover and bring to a boil. Reduce heat and cook slowly, stirring frequently, for 25 minutes or until potatoes are tender. Serve hot.

Serves 6

NUTRITIVE VALUES PER SERVING:

FAT	FIBER	VIT. A	VIT. C	CAL	CAL FROM FAT
2.52gm	5.60gm	495 IU	51.8mg	116	20%

JULIENNE OF TURNIPS AND CARROTS

1 pound carrots
1 pound turnips (or rutabagas)
2 teaspoons margarine
2 tablespoons broth
½ teaspoon salt
¼ teaspoon pepper
¼ teaspoon thyme

Cut carrots and turnips into 2-inch pieces, then cut each piece into matchstick-sized pieces. Steam vegetables until just tender, about 3 minutes. Drain well. May be done ahead and refrigerated at this point.

Just before serving, melt margarine with broth; toss vegetables gently with margarine-broth mixture to coat well. Season with salt, pepper, and thyme, heating thoroughly but not overcooking.

Serves 6

Nutritive Values per Serving:

FAT	FIBER	VIT. A	VIT. C	CAL	CAL FROM FAT
1.60gm	5.31gm	7993 IU	20.9mg	47.4	30%

LEMON BROCCOLI

2 bunches broccoli (about 2 pounds)
½ cup dry bread crumbs
1 teaspoon finely grated lemon peel
1 tablespoon margarine or butter
1 clove garlic, minced
½ teaspoon salt
⅛ teaspoon pepper
1 tablespoon fresh lemon juice
¼ cup chicken broth

Break broccoli into florets. Cut ends off stems and peel outside of stalks. Slice tender inside of stalks and place in steamer with florets. Steam broccoli florets and stems until almost tender.

In a nonstick skillet, heat crumbs over very low heat, stirring often, until a golden color. Remove crumbs from skillet and mix with lemon peel. Reserve. In the same skillet, melt margarine and sauté garlic over low heat until light golden. Add salt, pepper, lemon juice, and broth. Toss broccoli gently in mixture to coat. Transfer to baking dish and top with crumbs. Bake in a preheated 300°F oven for 5–10 minutes, or until hot. Don't overcook.

Serves 6

NUTRITIVE VALUES PER SERVING:

FAT	FIBER	VIT. A	VIT. C	CAL	CAL FROM FAT
2.80gm	9.21gm	3864 IU	138mg	83.7	30%

MARINATED CARROTS

2 tablespoons broth
2 teaspoons red wine vinegar
2 teaspoons olive oil
2 garlic cloves
⅛ teaspoon white pepper
¼ teaspoon salt
1½ teaspoons sugar
½ cup chopped fresh watercress
1½ pounds carrots

Combine all ingredients except carrots to make marinade. Slice carrots and steam until barely fork-tender. Drain carrots well and add to marinade. Marinate several hours or overnight. Serve chilled, or heat gently and serve as a hot vegetable.

Serves 8

NUTRITIVE VALUES PER SERVING:

FAT	FIBER	VIT. A	VIT. C	CAL	CAL FROM FAT
1.29gm	3.76gm	8983 IU	5.73mg	34.7	33%

MUSTARD CREAM BROCCOLI AND CARROTS

1 pound carrots, cut into long sticks

2 cups chicken broth

1 pound broccoli stems, peeled and cut into long sticks*

3 tablespoons low-fat yogurt

3 tablespoons of reserved broth from cooking vegetables

1 teaspoon dijon mustard

1 teaspoon fresh lemon juice

½ teaspoon salt

¼ teaspoon pepper

½ teaspoon sugar

2 tablespoons finely chopped fresh watercress

2 tablespoons finely chopped scallions

Simmer carrots in 2 cups broth for 5 minutes. Remove with a slotted spoon. Simmer broccoli stems in same broth for 3 minutes. Drain, saving broth. Keep vegetables separate.

Mix remaining ingredients to make sauce. Marinate vegetables separately in sauce (half for each vegetable) for several hours. Serve chilled or at room temperature, alongside one another.

Serves 6

---

*This is a good use for the too-often discarded broccoli stems.

NUTRITIVE VALUES PER SERVING:

FAT	FIBER	VIT. A	VIT. C	CAL	CAL FROM FAT
.873gm	7.98gm	9909 IU	74.0mg	49.4	16%

ONIONS FILLED WITH SPINACH

8 medium-small onions, outer "paper" layer
   removed
1 tablespoon margarine or butter
1 10-ounce package frozen chopped spinach,
   defrosted and squeezed dry
1 teaspoon fresh lemon juice
½ teaspoon salt
¼ teaspoon pepper
3 tablespoons low-fat yogurt
2 tablespoons onion cooking liquid
1½ tablespoons madeira wine
4 tablespoons bread crumbs

Cut top quarter off stem end of onion (the root end holds the layers together). Boil, partly covered, 15 minutes. Lift from water carefully, reserving cooking liquid. Gently cut out the center, leaving about 4 outside layers. Inside layers may be saved for other uses. Be careful not to pierce through the bottom of the onion. Turn upside down to drain.

Melt margarine: add spinach and heat through. Add all remaining ingredients except bread crumbs: blend together and cook over low heat for 5 minutes. Divide filling among onion shells and sprinkle each with ½ tablespoon bread crumbs. Bake in a preheated 350°F oven for 20 minutes. If made ahead and refrigerated, increase baking time to 30 minutes.

Serves 8

NUTRITIVE VALUES PER SERVING:

FAT	FIBER	VIT. A	VIT. C	CAL	CAL FROM FAT
1.88gm	3.69gm	3188 IU	18.8mg	74.7	23%

OVEN FRENCH FRIES

2 pounds unpeeled potatoes
2 tablespoons corn or safflower oil
½ teaspoon pepper
½ teaspoon paprika

Cut potatoes into large sticks. In a large bowl, toss potato sticks with oil, pepper, and paprika to coat thoroughly. Place potato sticks on a nonstick baking pan in a single layer. Bake for 20 minutes in a preheated 375°F oven. Loosen fries with a spatula and gently toss. Bake 20 minutes more, loosen with spatula, and serve.

Serves 6

NUTRITIVE VALUES PER SERVING:

FAT	FIBER	VIT. A	VIT. C	CAL	CAL FROM FAT
4.73gm	4.26gm	.99 IU	30.0mg	181	24%

RATATOUILLE

2 small eggplants, peeled
2 tablespoons olive oil
4 small zucchini, sliced
2 cups chopped onions
3 cloves garlic, minced
3 green peppers, cut into cubes
2 cups chopped tomatoes
1 teaspoon oregano
½ cup chopped fresh parsley
½ teaspoon salt
¼ teaspoon pepper
½ teaspoon sugar
6 cups cooked brown rice

Slice eggplants thinly, sprinkle with salt, and drain in colander for 30 minutes. Pat dry. Brush a nonstick skillet with a little of the oil. Sauté eggplant slices over medium heat until softened, brushing skillet with a bit more oil as needed. Set aside. Add remaining oil and sauté zucchini slices. Lift out with a slotted spoon and set aside. In the oil left in pan, sauté onions and garlic for 5 minutes over medium heat. Add peppers, tomatoes, oregano, parsley, salt, pepper, and sugar. Cook 5 minutes more.

In a casserole with a cover, arrange half the eggplant slices, then half the zucchini, then half the tomato mixture. Repeat layers with other half of eggplant, zucchini, and tomato mixture. Bake, covered, for 1 hour in a preheated 325°F oven.

As Ratatouille bakes, start rice, cooking according to package directions. Keep rice warm until Ratatouille is done. Serve Ratatouille over rice.

Serves 8

Nutritive Values per Serving:

FAT	FIBER	VIT. A	VIT. C	CAL	CAL FROM FAT
5.14gm	11.0gm	1485 IU	92.1mg	273	17%

ROMANIAN
VEGETABLE CASSEROLE

1 cup thinly sliced carrots
1 cup fresh green beans, sliced into ½-inch
   pieces
1 cup diced potatoes
2 medium tomatoes, cut into quarters
1 medium red onion, thinly sliced
1 cup diced rutabaga or turnip
½ head cauliflower, broken into small florets
½ cup chopped green and/or red bell pepper
1 cup peas, fresh or frozen
1 cup vegetable or chicken broth
1 tablespoon olive oil
3 cloves garlic, minced
½ teaspoon salt
¼ teaspoon thyme
¼ teaspoon basil
½ teaspoon oregano
¼ teaspoon pepper

Gently toss carrots, beans, potatoes, tomatoes, onion, rutabaga, cauliflower, peppers, and peas together and place in ungreased 9″ × 13″ baking pan. Combine broth, oil, garlic, and seasonings in a pan and heat to boiling. Pour broth mixture over vegetables. Cover pan with a tight lid or heavy foil.

Bake about 35–45 minutes in a preheated 350°F oven. Cook only until vegetables are tender. Stir once or twice during cooking process, so vegetables cook evenly. Serve hot.

Serves 6

NUTRITIVE VALUES PER SERVING:

FAT	FIBER	VIT. A	VIT. C	CAL	CAL FROM FAT
2.79gm	8.47gm	3441 IU	81.3mg	100	25%

SCALLOPED POTATOES AND CARROTS

2 cups carrots, sliced
¼ teaspoon salt
½ cup chopped scallions
2 pounds potatoes, sliced thinly (peeled)
¼ teaspoon salt (additional)
¼ teaspoon pepper
6 tablespoons parmesan cheese
2 tablespoons cold margarine, cut into small
   pieces
1½ cups low-fat milk
5 tablespoons nonfat dry milk

Steam carrots until barely done. Drain and toss with ¼ teaspoon salt and scallions. Coat a large casserole dish with cooking spray. Making 3 layers, arrange ⅓ of potatoes, then ⅓ of carrot mixture, seasoning each layer with ⅓ salt, pepper, parmesan, and dots of cold margarine. End layers with dots of margarine. Whisk low-fat milk with nonfat dry milk to combine. Pour over vegetables and bake for 1 hour in a preheated 350°F oven, covered with foil or a tight-fitting lid. Remove cover, baste well with liquid, and bake 30 minutes longer.

Serves 6

NUTRITIVE VALUES PER SERVING:

FAT	FIBER	VIT. A	VIT. C	CAL	CAL FROM FAT
6.65gm	6.66gm	5891 IU	35.0mg	250	24%

SOUTHERN GREENS AND TURNIPS

½ pound fresh mustard greens, coarsely chopped
3 medium turnips or rutabagas, chopped into
    small pieces
2 teaspoons corn or safflower oil
1 tablespoon broth
1 cup chopped onion
½ teaspoon sugar
½ teaspoon salt
⅛ teaspoon cayenne pepper

Wash greens and steam until just wilted; drain. Steam turnips until fork tender, and drain. Heat oil and broth and sauté onion until soft. Add turnips, greens, sugar, salt, and cayenne to onion mixture and heat through, tossing to combine well. Serve hot.

Serves 6

NUTRITIVE VALUES PER SERVING:

FAT	FIBER	VIT. A	VIT. C	CAL	CAL FROM FAT
1.99gm	5.33gm	2205 IU	46.4mg	58.2	31%

SPECIALLY SEASONED TOMATOES

12 medium tomatoes
2 tablespoons margarine or butter
2 tablespoons vegetable broth
1 teaspoon salt
¼ teaspoon pepper
1½ teaspoons garlic powder
1½ tablespoons ground cumin
1½ tablespoons ground coriander
1½ cups cornflake crumbs
½ cup finely chopped parsley

Place tomatoes stem end down, and cut off the top quarter (use tops in salads or other dishes). Soften margarine and mix well with broth. Add remaining ingredients and combine thoroughly.

Divide cornflake mixture among the 12 tomatoes: round mixture with hands to replace top quarter of tomato that was cut off. Chill for 1 hour.

Bake for 30 minutes in a preheated 300°F oven. Allow to set for 10 minutes before serving.

Serves 12

NUTRITIVE VALUES PER SERVING:

FAT	FIBER	VIT. A	VIT. C	CAL	CAL FROM FAT
2.13gm	2.71gm	1582 IU	34.4mg	58.7	33%

SPINACH-FILLED TOMATOES

8 medium-small tomatoes
1 tablespoon margarine
1 tablespoon flour
½ cup low-fat milk
1 10-ounce package frozen chopped spinach,
    defrosted and squeezed dry
½ teaspoon salt
¼ teaspoon pepper
4 tablespoons bread crumbs

Place tomatoes stem side down and cut off the top quarter (reserve tops for other uses). Carefully scoop out pulp, being cautious not to pierce sides or bottom. Turn upside down to drain.

Melt margarine and add flour; cook until golden. Add milk, blend, and cook until thickened. Add spinach, salt, and pepper and heat through. Fill tomatoes and sprinkle each with ½ tablespoon bread crumbs. Bake for 20 minutes in a preheated 350°F oven.

Serves 8

NUTRITIVE VALUES PER SERVING:

FAT	FIBER	VIT. A	VIT. C	CAL	CAL FROM FAT
2.20gm	4.34gm	4280 IU	35.5mg	73.7	27%

SPINACH PANCAKES

These are wonderful plain, or may be served with Dill Sauce,
Creamy Mustard Dressing (see Index), or a spoonful of yogurt.

1¾ cups low-fat milk
½ teaspoon salt
⅛ teaspoon nutmeg
¼ teaspoon pepper
1 cup unbleached white flour
1½ tablespoons margarine or butter, melted and
    cooled
2 eggs
½ teaspoon sugar
2 10-ounce packages frozen chopped spinach,
    defrosted and squeezed dry

In a blender, combine milk, salt, nutmeg, pepper, and flour; add melted margarine and blend again. Add eggs and sugar and blend well. Add spinach and blend just until combined; don't process more than necessary.

Cover the bottom of a heavy skillet with cooking spray and set skillet over medium heat until it is hot. For each pancake, drop 2 tablespoons of batter onto the skillet and spread batter out into a round pancake. Cook pancakes 2–3 minutes on each side, or until they have browned lightly. Keep hot on a warm platter, covered loosely with foil. Add more cooking spray to the skillet as needed to cook the remaining pancakes.

Serves 8

NUTRITIVE VALUES PER SERVING:

FAT	FIBER	VIT. A	VIT. C	CAL	CAL FROM FAT
4.93gm	4.95gm	6423 IU	15.3mg	141	31%

STIR-FRIED BROCCOLI

1 pound broccoli, stalks peeled and sliced
1 teaspoon corn or safflower oil
1 tablespoon chicken broth
1 clove garlic, minced
6 tablespoons chicken broth (additional)
1½ teaspoons soy sauce
1 tablespoon cornstarch
1 tablespoon water

Break broccoli into small florets and add to sliced stalks. Heat oil and 1 tablespoon chicken broth to high. Add broccoli and minced garlic to oil and broth and fry, tossing constantly, for 2 minutes. Add the 6 tablespoons chicken broth and soy sauce, cover, and let simmer for 3 minutes. Uncover, bring to a boil, add cornstarch mixed with water, and stir until thickened—about 1 minute. Serve hot.

Serves 4

NUTRITIVE VALUES PER SERVING:

FAT	FIBER	VIT. A	VIT. C	CAL	CAL FROM FAT
1.61gm	6.90gm	2842 IU	102mg	44.1	33%

STUFFED WHITE POTATOES

6 medium baking potatoes
2 tablespoons margarine or butter, at room
    temperature
2 tablespoons chicken broth
4 tablespoons low-fat milk
4 tablespoons part-skim ricotta cheese
½ teaspoon salt
¼ teaspoon pepper
3 tablespoons bread crumbs
6 tablespoons sliced scallions

Bake potatoes in a preheated 375°F oven for 45 minutes to 1 hour, until done. Cut a lengthwise slice off each potato and scoop out most of the potato center, leaving enough to support the shell. Whip the potato centers with margarine, broth, milk, ricotta, salt, and pepper.

Mix bread crumbs and sliced scallions together. Fill shells with potato mixture and sprinkle each potato with 1½ tablespoons of bread crumb–scallion mixture. Bake at 375°F for 25 minutes or until heated through.

Serves 6

NUTRITIVE VALUES PER SERVING:

FAT	FIBER	VIT. A	VIT. C	CAL	CAL FROM FAT
5.17gm	4.60gm	348 IU	33.1mg	213	22%

SWEET AND TART LENTILS

2 cups dried lentils
2 tablespoons corn or safflower oil
½ cup chopped onion
1 clove garlic, minced
2 tablespoons red wine vinegar
1 cup chicken or vegetable broth
1 tablespoon cornstarch
2 tablespoons sugar
¼ teaspoon nutmeg
½ teaspoon salt
¼ teaspoon pepper

Simmer lentils in enough water to cover for 30 minutes. Drain lentils and keep warm.

Heat oil in a large skillet; add onion and garlic and sauté until softened. Combine vinegar with broth, cornstarch, sugar, nutmeg, salt, and pepper and add to onion mixture. Cook until thickened, stirring constantly. Add lentils to onion mixture and mix well, stirring gently so lentils don't get mushy. Serve hot.

Serves 6

NUTRITIVE VALUES PER SERVING:

FAT	FIBER	VIT. A	VIT. C	CAL	CAL FROM FAT
5.44gm	7.70gm	49.7 IU	5.76mg	274	18%

SWEET POTATO
AND CARROT MOLD

The center of this vegetable mold may be filled with another vegetable such as broccoli, sautéed cherry tomatoes, or peas for a dramatic color contrast.

1 pound carrots
1 pound sweet potatoes
1 cup chopped onion
2 tablespoons margarine or butter
2 egg whites, unbeaten
2 garlic cloves, minced
¼ teaspoon thyme
½ cup bread crumbs
1 cup low-fat milk
1 teaspoon celery salt
½ teaspoon pepper
2 tablespoons fresh lemon juice
½ cup chopped fresh parsley

Slice carrots. Peel, quarter, and slice sweet potatoes to the same thickness as carrots. Bring 4 cups of water to a boil. Add carrots and sweet potatoes and bring to a second boil. Cover and simmer 10–15 minutes, just until barely tender. Drain well and mash (save cooking liquid for other uses).

Sauté onions in margarine for 5 minutes. Add to mashed vegetables and mix in all other ingredients except parsley. Pack into a 4-cup ring mold or other ovenproof dish sprayed lightly with cooking spray. Place ring mold into a baking pan with one inch of hot water in bottom. Bake, uncovered, in a preheated 350°F oven for 1 hour.

Remove mold from baking pan and loosen vegetable mixture from sides and bottom of mold with a metal spatula. Invert onto a serving plate and slip mold off vegetable ring. Sprinkle with parsley and serve.

Serves 8

Nutritive Values per Serving:

FAT	FIBER	VIT. A	VIT. C	CAL	CAL FROM FAT
4.26gm	5.52gm	11,366 IU	27.7mg	177	22%

SWEET POTATO FRIES

These are an especially delicious and colorful addition to meals with poultry and veal. They do hold their shape, but do not expect them to be crispy.

**1 pound unpeeled sweet potatoes, cut into large
  sticks
1½ tablespoons corn or safflower oil
½ teaspoon salt**

Toss potato sticks with oil, then sprinkle with salt and toss to coat all potato sticks evenly with salt and oil. Place potato sticks in a single layer on a nonstick pan. Bake for 20 minutes in a pre-heated 350°F oven. Turn with a metal spatula and bake an additional 20 minutes.

Serves 4

Nutritive Values per Serving:

FAT	FIBER	VIT. A	VIT. C	CAL	CAL FROM FAT
5.85gm	4.07gm	9181 IU	24.8mg	204	26%

SWEET POTATO PANCAKES

These pancakes are fine by themselves, or may be topped with low-fat yogurt and green onions or with applesauce.

1 cup grated white potato (peeling is optional)
1 cup grated sweet potato (peeling is optional)
1 cup grated carrots
3 beaten eggs
⅓ cup flour
¼ teaspoon salt
1 tablespoon fresh lemon juice
2 tablespoons finely chopped onion
¼ cup chopped fresh parsley

Place grated potatoes in a colander; salt lightly and let drain for 15 minutes. Rinse and squeeze out all the liquid (save liquid for soups or other uses). Combine potatoes with remaining ingredients and stir to mix well.

Coat griddle or skillet with cooking spray. Use 2 tablespoons batter for each pancake. Fry pancakes over medium heat until golden brown and crisp on both sides. Serve immediately.

Serves 6

NUTRITIVE VALUES PER SERVING:

FAT	FIBER	VIT. A	VIT. C	CAL	CAL FROM FAT
3.07gm	3.04gm	4596 IU	16.6mg	124	22%

SWEET POTATO-RICE BAKE

3 tablespoons margarine or butter, melted and
  cooled
1 cup chopped onion
1 cup chopped celery
1 cup brown rice, raw
2½ cups vegetable or chicken broth
½ teaspoon salt
½ teaspoon pepper
¼ teaspoon ground coriander
½ teaspoon thyme
⅛ teaspoon powdered ginger
2 eggs, beaten
1 17-ounce can sweet potatoes, drained and cut
  into small cubes

Heat margarine in skillet. Sauté onion, celery, and rice for 5
minutes. Add 2 cups of broth, salt, pepper, coriander, thyme, and
ginger. Bring to boiling; reduce heat and simmer, covered, for 40
minutes. Transfer rice mixture to a dish and let cool.

Beat eggs with remaining ½ cup broth. Blend into cooled rice
mixture. Add sweet potato cubes. Toss together gently, combining well. Place in a casserole lightly coated with cooking spray
and bake in preheated 350°F oven for 30 minutes. If prepared
ahead and refrigerated, bake 40 minutes.

Serves 8

NUTRITIVE VALUES PER SERVING:

FAT	FIBER	VIT. A	VIT. C	CAL	CAL FROM FAT
7.00gm	4.77gm	5188 IU	16.3mg	241	26%

SWEET POTATOES WITH APPLES

4 large sweet potatoes or yams, quartered
½ cup brown sugar
¼ cup orange juice
2 teaspoons grated orange rind
½ teaspoon cinnamon
2 large, tart unpeeled cooking apples, sliced
2 tablespoons margarine or butter, chilled and
    cut into small pieces

Simmer sweet potatoes in water for about 20 minutes or until just tender. Drain, cool slightly, and slice ½ inch thick. Combine brown sugar, orange juice, orange rind, and cinnamon. Layer ⅓ of potato slices, ⅓ of apple slices, and sprinkle with ⅓ of orange-sugar mixture. Repeat layers twice until all ingredients are used. Dot top with margarine. Bake, uncovered, in a preheated 350°F oven for 30 minutes or until potatoes and apples are tender.

Serves 8

NUTRITIVE VALUES PER SERVING:

FAT	FIBER	VIT. A	VIT. C	CAL	CAL FROM FAT
3.44gm	3.46gm	5915 IU	20.7mg	198	16%

SWISS CHARD FRITTERS

These fritters may be served with a light white sauce (such as Thyme Sauce—see Index) or a tomato-type sauce, although they are absolutely delicious by themselves.

1 cup unbleached white flour
⅔ cup low-fat milk
2 eggs, beaten
1 tablespoon melted margarine or butter, cooled
2 cups fresh swiss chard leaves, chopped
1 onion, finely chopped
½ teaspoon salt
¼ teaspoon pepper

Combine all ingredients to make batter. Lightly coat a skillet or griddle with cooking spray and heat to medium. Use 2 table-spoons of batter for each fritter, pressing down on each mound of batter to flatten, and fry on each side until golden and slightly crisp. Repeat until all batter is used, adding cooking spray to skillet or griddle as needed.

Serves 6

NUTRITIVE VALUES PER SERVING:

FAT	FIBER	VIT. A	VIT. C	CAL	CAL FROM FAT
4.63gm	3.26gm	3382 IU	12.4mg	152	27%

WALNUT-STUFFED SWEET POTATOES

4 medium sweet potatoes, washed
1½ tablespoons margarine or butter
¼ cup orange juice
½ teaspoon salt
4 teaspoons finely chopped walnuts

Bake potatoes in a preheated 375°F oven for 45 minutes to 1 hour, until fork tender. Cut a long slice off the top of each potato and scoop out the center, leaving a ½-inch-thick shell. Whip potato centers with margarine, orange juice, and salt until light and fluffy. Spoon potato mixture back into shells. Sprinkle with walnuts. Bake at 375°F for 20 minutes, or until heated through.

Serves 4

NUTRITIVE VALUES PER SERVING:

FAT	FIBER	VIT. A	VIT. C	CAL	CAL FROM FAT
7.47gm	4.4gm	9438 IU	32.8mg	230	29%

WHITE BEANS

These beans are a delicious and unusual accompaniment to a roast or stew that has a sauce. Spoon a bit of sauce over each serving of beans, and omit olive oil in the recipe.

1 pound white beans
½ teaspoon salt
¼ teaspoon pepper
2 cloves garlic, minced
1 teaspoon basil
1 bunch fresh watercress, chopped
2 tablespoons olive oil

Cover beans with water and soak overnight. Drain. Cover again with water and bring to a boil. Cover pan and simmer 50–60 minutes, or until beans are tender (don't overcook). Drain beans and toss gently with salt, pepper, garlic, basil, watercress, and olive oil. Serve immediately.

Any leftovers can be served cold as a bean salad.

Serves 8

NUTRITIVE VALUES PER SERVING:

FAT	FIBER	VIT. A	VIT. C	CAL	CAL FROM FAT
4.29gm	2.58gm	199 IU	3.17mg	223	17%

WINTER VEGETABLE MEDLEY

6 medium red potatoes, cubed
6 medium carrots, sliced
12 ounces brussels sprouts, halved (fresh, or
   frozen and defrosted)
2 tablespoons margarine or butter
2 cloves garlic, minced
¼ cup sliced scallions
½ teaspoon thyme
½ teaspoon salt
¼ teaspoon pepper
¼ cup chopped fresh parsley

Steam potatoes and carrots for 10 minutes. Add sprouts and steam 10 minutes more, or until all vegetables are fork tender (don't overcook). Melt margarine in a large skillet and sauté garlic, scallions, thyme, salt, and pepper for 5 minutes. Add vegetables to margarine mixture and gently toss, heating thoroughly. Sprinkle with parsley and serve.

Serves 8

NUTRITIVE VALUES PER SERVING:

FAT	FIBER	VIT. A	VIT. C	CAL	CAL FROM FAT
3.21gm	7.17gm	6586 IU	62.3mg	136	21%

7
Pasta, Rice, Grains, and Breads

Apple-Oatmeal Cereal
Apricot Bread
Baked Rice
Baking Soda Biscuits
Barley Pilaf
Bran Muffins
Brazilian Rice
Carrot-Zucchini Bread
Chicken Fried Rice
Chilled Chinese Noodles
Corn Bread
Corn Bread Stuffing
Cornmeal with Honey
Corn Muffins
Curried Rice
Garlic Herb Bread
Green Chili Corn Bread

Green Rice
Lemon Rice
Maple Syrup Oatmeal
Parsley-Cheese Noodles
Pasta Shells with Peas
Pasta with Garlic and Watercress
Pasta with Peppers and Parmesan
Pilaf
Rice with Mushrooms
Risotto
Spanish Rice
Vermicelli-Rice Pilaf
Vermicelli with Broccoli
Whole-Wheat Biscuits
Whole-Wheat Bread Stuffing
Whole-Wheat Scones
Yorkshire Pudding

Pasta, Rice, Grains, and Breads

If you've ever driven through midwest America in the summer, you've seen a golden ocean—the "amber waves of grain" we sing about in "America the Beautiful." Wheat and corn fields literally blanket the Midwest, making this nation the largest producer of grain in the world. We produce it—why don't we eat it?

The American Cancer Society strongly recommends that we eat more whole grains. This chapter is designed to provide you with some wonderful recipes and a variety of uses for whole wheat, cornmeal, brown rice, bulgur, barley, and whole oats. Wait until you taste these!—Pasta Shells with Peas, Risotto, Pilaf, Golden Cornbread—all delicious and all made from vitamin- and fiber-rich whole ingredients.

When we talk about "whole foods" we mean food in an unprocessed state. Over the years—in the name of progress—we have bleached, refined, and stripped grains so they will look prettier and have a softer texture. But in exchange, we have depleted them of most of their original nutrients.

Let's begin with that staple American grain, wheat. The most wholesome breads and pastas made with this grain are made with *whole*-wheat flour. Anything less than the whole grain of the wheat cheats you of vitamins, minerals, and fiber. There are three parts to a kernel of wheat. The outer part is the *bran* and consists of six layers of "skin," primarily dietary fiber. The bran also contains B vitamins, iron, and other minerals. The second part of the wheat kernel is the *germ*, and is located in the heart of the kernel. It contains oil, carbohydrates, protein, vitamin E, B vitamins (especially thiamin), iron, and other minerals. The third part, the white center of the kernel, is the *endosperm*, which is primarily carbohydrates and starch and contains some protein.

If you buy *stone-ground whole-wheat* products, the bran, wheat germ, and endosperm are all preserved. If you buy white flour—especially bleached flour—the bran and wheat germ have been removed, eliminating B vitamins, minerals, and fiber. Although some flours are "enriched"—generally meaning that thiamin (B_1), riboflavin (B_2), niacin (B_3), and iron have been added back—most of the fiber, other B vitamins, other vitamins, and many minerals are still missing.

We know you can't use whole-wheat flour for everything—its texture is sometimes too coarse and grainy for fine pastries. But you can usually *combine* it with white flour for soft and delicious baked goods. If you have never baked with whole-wheat flour, you will find that it yields a tasty, hearty product. If your family is used to only white bread, start out by using a larger proportion of unbleached flour to whole-wheat flour and gradually reverse the flour proportions. Fresh hot Whole-Wheat Scones, Apricot Bread, Bran Muffins, and Baking Soda Biscuits will delight even the most skeptical member of the family.

Use whole-wheat pasta and noodles in all pasta recipes. Whole-wheat spaghetti, elbow macaroni, egg noodles, and shells are readily available in most supermarkets. If you can't find these products in your local market, try your local health food store. Whole-wheat pasta has a delicious taste and a truly al dente texture when cooked, is full of vitamins and fiber, and is generally preferable to any other kind of pasta. If you like to use "vegetable" pastas, read the package label to make sure that the vegetable is first or second on the ingredients list. Otherwise you are probably buying white pasta colored with vegetable dye.

Cornmeal is another grain that makes delicious bread and cereals and isn't used as much as it could be. Who can resist hot corn bread or cornmeal muffins? For interesting variety, try Green Chili Corn Bread with a hearty soup. It doesn't even need butter—it tastes scrumptious by itself. Or surprise your family with steaming Cornmeal with Honey instead of cold cereal on a chilly winter morning. When making dishes with cornmeal, use the whole, bolted varieties; they are more nutritious and contain almost three times the fiber of degermed cornmeal.

When was the last time you used rolled oats? You can do more
with oats than just plain oatmeal for breakfast. Remember those
soft, chewy oatmeal cookies in your lunchbox? We offer Peanut
Butter-Oatmeal Cookies as well as a delicious Oatmeal Cake (see
Index). Oatmeal for breakfast, in a recipe like Apple-Oatmeal
Cereal or Maple Syrup Oatmeal, is a tasty and nutritious way to
begin your day. Served with low-fat milk, it becomes a complete
low-fat protein. Oatmeal is fast and convenient, and lends itself
to innovation. Create your own taste treats with extras like
peaches, raisins, apples, a tablespoon of honey, a chopped date,
or dried apricots—the possibilities are endless. A warm bowl of
oatmeal with a little cinnamon and milk is also a great bedtime
snack. This inexpensive grain is a nutrient gold mine—eat it
often!

Rice, another excellent grain, is probably the most universal
food. Every country has its favorite rice dish. It is usually one of
the first foods (infant rice cereal) we give to babies. Steamed
rice, baked rice, fried rice, or herbed rice—it is a food that is
versatile, easy to cook, and suitable for any occasion. Rice comes
in three forms: brown or whole rice, white (polished) rice, and
parboiled or converted rice. Brown rice retains all the original
nutrients of the rice kernel. White or polished rice is stripped of
its outer layers and many of its vitamins, minerals, fiber, and
some protein. Parboiled or "converted" rice retains more of the
original nutrients because the process of parboiling pushes some
of the vitamins from the bran to the white endosperm.

Brown rice versus white rice—which is the best to use? Brown
rice does contain more fiber, vitamins, and minerals than white
rice. Nutritionally, brown rice wins right there. It also has a
thicker consistency and crunchier texture than white rice, which
makes it a welcome addition to many vegetarian dishes. The
taste is delicious and you feel you are eating real substance.
However, in some dishes, white rice is more aesthetically pleas-
ing to the eye than natural brown rice (Mandarin Rice Pudding
in the Desserts chapter is made with white rice). What we have
tried to do is make a variety of dishes with both kinds of rice.
Any of the dishes using brown rice can be made with white rice
and vice versa. Just be sure to change the cooking time: brown
rice takes longer to cook (see pages 189–190 for rice cooking
times). If the recipe calls for brown rice and you use white rice,
the fiber per serving will be less than the value given for that
recipe. With some popular rice dishes we have created two
varieties—one with white rice and one with brown. Risotto, for
example, uses brown rice. Rice with Mushrooms (also a risotto)
uses white rice.

Low-fat versions of rice recipe favorites include Baked Rice for an elegant dinner party, Chicken Fried Rice (which can also be a complete meal), Spanish Rice, and Curried Rice. Vermicelli-Rice Pilaf combines two grains and is a wonderful complement for chicken or fish dishes.

Brazilian Rice—a mixture of vegetables, rice, and cheese—is another versatile dish that can be made into a complete meal by adding cooked cubes of chicken or turkey. Remember never to overcook rice; it becomes mushy.

Try these exciting and unusual grain recipes:

- For lovers of Oriental food, Chilled Chinese Noodles is a perfect buffet dish. Flavored with a bit of sesame, peanut, and hot chili oil, its taste is both subtle and authentically piquant. Serve with poultry or fish.
- Rice with Mushrooms is made with dried porcini mushrooms soaked in dry white wine and served with parmesan cheese—a wonderful side dish to serve with any Northern Italian entrée using chicken or seafood.
- Parsley-Cheese Noodles is a casserole dish using cottage cheese, with a bit of feta for flavor and melt-in-your-mouth texture, and carrots to add vitamins and lively color. This can also be served as a light entrée.
- Vermicelli with Broccoli and Pasta Shells with Peas are two unusual pasta dishes that could either be a side dish or a first course at a dinner party.
- Both Pasta with Garlic and Watercress and Pasta with Peppers and Parmesan derive their distinctive flavors from fresh garlic and ripe bell pepper. They are wonderful side dishes for blander entrées like poached fish or poultry.

The fat content in most of our pasta, rice, and grain dishes is below 30% calories from fat. For those dishes slightly above 30%, follow the general rule given for vegetables: *fancy entrée/plain side dish or vegetable.*

COOKING METHODS
When Is Bread Done?

Many ovens do not perform true to temperature and cooking times. To determine if breads or muffins are done, try these tests:

- Pierce the center of the product with a toothpick: if it comes out clean the bread.or muffin is done.
- Gently touch the center of the product with your finger: if it springs back instead of leaving an indent, the bread or muffin is done.

Cooking Perfect Pasta

Bring slightly salted water to a rapid boil in a large pot over high heat (the water will take about ten minutes to reach a rapid boil). Add a few drops of olive oil to help prevent the pasta from sticking, and to prevent the water from foaming over. Add the pasta a little at a time. When all the pasta is in the pot, stir with a fork to separate it, and let the water come back to a boil. Stir often to make sure the pasta doesn't stick together. Cooking time will vary depending on the size and thickness of the pasta. Thin pasta like vermicelli needs to boil for about five minutes. Thicker pasta like shells, eight to ten minutes. Pasta should be cooked al dente—slightly chewy. To test for doneness, let a piece cool and then pinch or bite it. The pasta should be slightly resistant, yet flexible. Drain the pasta in a large colander, briskly shaking to eliminate all excess moisture. It is important that the pasta be as dry as possible before topping with sauce. Nothing ruins a pasta dish more than water seeping out from the edges of the pasta and diluting the sauce. An easy way to reheat leftover plain pasta (in case you cooked too much): heat a large pot of water to rapid boiling. Put pasta in a metal sieve. Dunk into the water for about ten seconds and then drain. The pasta will be warmed but not mushy from overcooking.

APPLE-OATMEAL CEREAL

2 cups low-fat milk

2 tablespoons brown sugar

1 tablespoon margarine or butter

$\frac{1}{4}$ teaspoon salt

$\frac{1}{4}$ teaspoon cinnamon

1 cup rolled oats

1 cup chopped unpeeled apples

$\frac{1}{2}$ cup raisins

$\frac{1}{4}$ cup brown sugar for garnish

1 cup low-fat milk (additional)

Combine 2 cups milk, 2 tablespoons brown sugar, margarine, salt, cinnamon, oats, apples, and raisins in a saucepan and bring to a boil. Simmer for 15 minutes, uncovered. Cover and let stand off heat 5 minutes before serving. Sprinkle each serving with 1 tablespoon brown sugar and pour on ¼ cup milk.

Serves 4

NUTRITIVE VALUES PER SERVING:

FAT	FIBER	VIT. A	VIT. C	CAL	CAL FROM FAT
6.71gm	3.67gm	394 IU	3.40mg	267	23%

APRICOT BREAD

2 cups whole-wheat flour
½ cup brown sugar
2 teaspoons baking soda
¼ teaspoon salt
1 teaspoon cinnamon
2 pounds fresh apricots, or 2 16-ounce cans, drained
2 eggs, slightly beaten
¼ cup corn or safflower oil
2 teaspoons vanilla

Mix dry ingredients together. Puree fresh or canned apricots in blender. Mix pureed apricots with eggs, oil, and vanilla, and add to dry mixture, blending well. Don't overmix, or loaf may be heavy. Coat a standard-sized loaf pan with cooking spray and flour. Scoop batter into loaf pan and bake for 55 minutes in a preheated 350°F. Cool a few minutes before removing from pan.

Serves 12

NUTRITIVE VALUES PER SERVING:

FAT	FIBER	VIT. A	VIT. C	CAL	CAL FROM FAT
7.31gm	4.20gm	2422 IU	9.07mg	229	29%

BAKED RICE

2 cups chicken broth
2 tablespoons margarine or butter
2 scallions, sliced
¼ teaspoon salt
¼ teaspoon pepper
1 cup raw white rice
¾ cup chopped fresh parsley

Preheat oven to 375°F.

Bring chicken broth to a boil; cover and keep warm until needed. Melt margarine over medium-high heat. Add scallions and cook until soft. Add salt and pepper. Reduce heat to medium; add rice and cook for 5 minutes. Carefully pour boiling broth into rice mixture; add parsley, cover, and put in the middle of the preheated oven. Bake at 375°F for 20 minutes, or until liquid is absorbed and the rice fluffy.

Serves 4

NUTRITIVE VALUES PER SERVING:

FAT	FIBER	VIT. A	VIT. C	CAL	CAL FROM FAT
6.74gm	2.49gm	1461 IU	23.3mg	240	25%

BAKING SODA BISCUITS

1 cup unbleached white flour
1 cup whole-wheat flour
½ teaspoon baking soda
¼ teaspoon salt
¼ cup margarine or butter
¾ cup buttermilk
1 tablespoon sesame seeds

Sift flours, baking soda, and salt into a large bowl. Using a fork or pastry blender, cut in margarine until mixture is crumbly. Add all the buttermilk at once and stir to make a soft dough.

Turn dough onto a lightly floured board and knead about five times, until mixture becomes a smooth ball. Roll to ½-inch thickness and cut with a 2½-inch cookie cutter, or shape with hands into 12 biscuits. Sprinkle with sesame seeds. Place on ungreased baking sheet; bake about 12 minutes in a preheated 450°F oven until lightly browned.

Makes 12 biscuits

NUTRITIVE VALUES PER BISCUIT:

FAT	FIBER	VIT. A	VIT. C	CAL	CAL FROM FAT
4.58gm	1.32gm	162 IU	.16mg	116	36%

BARLEY PILAF

½ cup sliced scallions
1½ tablespoons margarine or butter
1 cup barley, rinsed well in water and drained
2 cups chicken broth
½ teaspoon thyme
¼ teaspoon salt
¼ teaspoon pepper
¼ cup chopped cashews
¼ cup chopped fresh parsley

Sauté scallions in margarine for 5 minutes. Add barley, chicken broth, thyme, salt, pepper, and cashews. Bring to a boil, cover, and simmer 40–50 minutes or until tender. Sprinkle with parsley before serving.

Serves 6

NUTRITIVE VALUES PER SERVING:

FAT	FIBER	VIT. A	VIT. C	CAL	CAL FROM FAT
6.31gm	3.15gm	510 IU	6.99mg	181	31%

BRAN MUFFINS

½ cup whole-wheat flour
1½ cups unbleached white flour
1 cup 100% bran cereal
¼ cup wheat germ
1 tablespoon baking powder
1 teaspoon baking soda
½ teaspoon salt
1 tablespoon cinnamon
½ cup brown sugar
1 cup low-fat yogurt
½ cup low-fat milk
1 egg, slightly beaten
¼ cup honey
2 tablespoons corn or safflower oil
1 8-ounce can crushed pineapple in juice,
     undrained
2 cups raisins (optional)

Combine dry ingredients. Mix yogurt, milk, egg, honey, oil, pineapple and its juice, and raisins and add to dry ingredients. Combine well.

Coat muffin tins with cooking spray. Divide mixture to fill 24 muffin cups. Bake for 25 minutes in a preheated 400°F oven. Let cool a few minutes and remove from pan.

Makes 24 muffins

NUTRITIVE VALUES PER MUFFIN:

FAT	FIBER	VIT. A	VIT. C	CAL	CAL FROM FAT
1.94gm	2.24gm	32.1 IU	1.51mg	131	13%

BRAZILIAN RICE

½ pound fresh mushrooms, sliced
½ cup chopped onions
1 cup finely chopped cabbage
½ cup grated carrots
1 clove garlic, minced
3 tablespoons olive oil
1 6-ounce can tomato paste
½ teaspoon salt
¼ teaspoon pepper
½ teaspoon basil
⅛ teaspoon celery seed
1½ cups raw brown rice

Sauté mushrooms, onions, cabbage, carrots, and garlic in 1½ tablespoons of olive oil for 10 minutes. Add tomato paste, salt, pepper, basil, celery seed, and ⅓ cup water. Cover and simmer for 20 minutes. Sauté rice in remaining 1½ tablespoons oil until lightly browned. Add 3 cups hot water. Cover and simmer for 30 minutes. Add cooked vegetable mixture and simmer for 10 minutes, or until rice is tender.

Serves 8

NUTRITIVE VALUES PER SERVING:

FAT	FIBER	VIT. A	VIT. C	CAL	CAL FROM FAT
6.11gm	5.04gm	1743 IU	7.05mg	201	27%

CARROT-ZUCCHINI BREAD

½ cup whole-wheat flour
1½ cups unbleached white flour
1½ teaspoons cinnamon
1½ teaspoons baking powder
¼ teaspoon salt
¼ teaspoon allspice
⅔ cup brown sugar
¼ cup corn or safflower oil
2 teaspoons vanilla
2 whole eggs
½ cup low-fat milk
1⅓ cups grated carrots
⅔ cup grated zucchini

Combine dry ingredients. Mix oil, vanilla, eggs, and milk in blender or processor until blended. Add grated carrots and zucchini to oil mixture and blend for a few seconds, just until combined. Mix thoroughly with dry ingredients, but just until blended.

Pour into a loaf pan coated with cooking spray and bake in a preheated 350°F oven for 45–55 minutes, or until a cake tester (or toothpick) inserted into the center comes out clean. Cool for a few minutes and turn out of pan.

Serves 12

Nutritive Values per Serving:

FAT	FIBER	VIT. A	VIT. C	CAL	CAL FROM FAT
5.82gm	2.02gm	1904 IU	2.21mg	181	29%

CHICKEN FRIED RICE

½ cup grated carrots
1 cup chopped cooked chicken
1½ tablespoons oil
2 eggs, lightly beaten
½ teaspoon pepper
3 cups cooked brown rice (about 1 cup raw)
3 tablespoons soy sauce
⅔ cup sliced scallions

Sauté carrots and chicken in oil for 1 minute over medium heat, stirring constantly. Add eggs and pepper and cook over medium heat for 1 minute, stirring constantly. Add rice and soy sauce and fry for 5 minutes, stirring often. Garnish with sliced scallions. Serve immediately.

Serves 6

NUTRITIVE VALUES PER SERVING:

FAT	FIBER	VIT. A	VIT. C	CAL	CAL FROM FAT
6.93gm	3.16gm	1672 IU	4.32mg	219	29%

CHILLED CHINESE NOODLES

¾ pound whole-wheat vermicelli noodles (white
    may be substituted)
1 tablespoon sesame oil
3 tablespoons sliced scallions
1 cup grated carrots
½ tablespoon peanut oil
½ tablespoon hot chili oil (found in Oriental
    section of market)
3 tablespoons soy sauce
1 tablespoon red wine vinegar
1 tablespoon sugar

Cook vermicelli until tender, about 10 minutes. Drain, rinse
under cold water, and drain again. Toss with sesame oil and
reserve. Combine scallions, carrots, peanut oil, chili oil, soy
sauce, vinegar, and sugar. Toss with noodles. Let set for at least
1 hour to blend flavors. Serve at room temperature or chilled.

Serves 8

NUTRITIVE VALUES PER SERVING:

FAT	FIBER	VIT. A	VIT. C	CAL	CAL FROM FAT
4.13gm	5.76gm	2082 IU	1.87mg	214	17%

CORN BREAD

1 cup yellow cornmeal
1 cup unbleached white flour
1 tablespoon baking powder
3 tablespoons sugar
½ teaspoon salt
1 egg, beaten
1 cup low-fat milk
3 tablespoons corn oil

Combine cornmeal, flour, baking powder, sugar, and salt. Beat egg, milk, and oil together and add to dry ingredients. Mix just until all ingredients are combined. Pour batter into a loaf pan coated with cooking spray, and bake for 35 minutes in a pre-heated 350°F. Cool slightly before cutting.

Serves 12

NUTRITIVE VALUES PER SERVING:

FAT	FIBER	VIT. A	VIT. C	CAL	CAL FROM FAT
4.49gm	.64gm	114 IU	.19mg	139	29%

CORN BREAD STUFFING

3 tablespoons margarine or butter
1 cup chopped celery
¼ cup chopped onion
¼ cup chopped fresh parsley
½ cup water
3 cups coarse corn bread crumbs
3 cups dry bread crumbs (whole wheat, if available)
½ teaspoon poultry seasoning
1 cup chicken broth

Melt margarine and sauté celery, onion, and parsley for 10 minutes. Add water, cover, and cook for 5 minutes. Remove vegetable mixture from heat and toss with crumbs, poultry seasoning, and broth. Bake for 30 minutes in a preheated 350°F oven or fill an 8-pound turkey just before baking.

Serves 8/Stuffs an 8-pound turkey

NUTRITIVE VALUES PER SERVING:

FAT	FIBER	VIT. A	VIT. C	CAL	CAL FROM FAT
9.69gm	4.60gm	496 IU	4.70mg	301	29%

CORNMEAL WITH HONEY

1¼ cups yellow cornmeal
1 cup cold water
2 cups boiling water
½ teaspoon salt
¼ cup honey
½ cup low-fat milk

Combine cornmeal with 1 cup cold water. Bring 2 cups of water to a boil and gradually add cornmeal mixture. Add salt and cook for 20 minutes, stirring often. Serve with honey and milk.

Serves 4

NUTRITIVE VALUES PER SERVING:

FAT	FIBER	VIT. A	VIT. C	CAL	CAL FROM FAT
1.11gm	1.25gm	253 IU	.48mg	236	4%

CORN MUFFINS

1 cup yellow cornmeal
1½ cups unbleached white flour
¼ cup sugar
1 tablespoon baking powder
½ teaspoon salt
1½ cups low-fat milk
¼ cup corn oil
2 eggs, lightly beaten

Mix dry ingredients together. Beat milk, oil, and eggs together and mix with dry ingredients. Stir together just until combined— don't overmix. Spray 18 muffin cups with cooking spray and pour batter into cups. Bake for 20–25 minutes in a preheated 400°F oven.

Makes 18 muffins

NUTRITIVE VALUES PER MUFFIN:

FAT	FIBER	VIT. A	VIT. C	CAL	CAL FROM FAT
4.22gm	.53gm	104 IU	.19mg	122	31%

CURRIED RICE

3 cups cooked white rice (about 1 cup
   uncooked)
½ cup chopped celery
½ cup finely chopped onion
½ cup chopped fresh mushrooms
2 tablespoons margarine or butter
1½ tablespoons curry powder (or 1 tablespoon
   for milder flavor)
½ cup chutney, with large pieces chopped

Sauté celery, onions, and mushrooms in margarine until onions
are limp. Stir in curry powder and continue stirring for several
seconds until mixture is a golden color. Add chutney and cooked
rice. Toss gently to combine all ingredients and heat thoroughly
over low heat.

Serves 8

NUTRITIVE VALUES PER SERVING:

FAT	FIBER	VIT. A	VIT. C	CAL	CAL FROM FAT
3.05gm	1.33gm	148 IU	2.09mg	154	18%

GARLIC HERB BREAD

1 loaf whole-wheat french bread (white may be
    substituted)
2 tablespoons plus 2 teaspoons margarine or
    butter
4 cloves garlic, minced
5 tablespoons chicken broth
1 cup chopped parsley
¼ teaspoon oregano
¼ teaspoon thyme
¼ teaspoon basil
½ cup parmesan cheese, freshly grated
Paprika

Split bread lengthwise. Soften margarine. Using a fork, mix margarine with garlic until fluffy. Add broth, parsley, herbs, and cheese and blend thoroughly. Spread on bread halves and sprinkle each half with paprika. Bake for 10 minutes in a preheated 400°F oven.

Serves 10

NUTRITIVE VALUES PER SERVING:

FAT	FIBER	VIT. A	VIT. C	CAL	CAL FROM FAT
5.98gm	3.17gm	665 IU	10.3mg	174	31%

GREEN CHILI CORN BREAD

1 cup cornmeal
⅓ cup unbleached white flour
1 tablespoon brown sugar
½ teaspoon salt
2 teaspoons baking soda
⅓ cup nonfat dry milk
2 eggs, beaten
¾ cup warm water
2 tablespoons corn or safflower oil
1 4-ounce can diced green chilies, drained
3 ounces part-skim mozzarella cheese, grated
⅓ cup sliced scallions
1½ cups corn, frozen or canned, drained

Mix dry ingredients. Beat eggs, water, and oil together. Add chilies, cheese, scallions, and corn to liquid mixture. Add dry ingredients to liquid mixture and stir until thoroughly combined. Pour into a loaf pan lightly coated with cooking spray. Bake for 30 minutes in a preheated 425°F oven.

Serves 12

NUTRITIVE VALUES PER SERVING:

FAT	FIBER	VIT. A	VIT. C	CAL	CAL FROM FAT
4.67gm	1.86gm	365 IU	8.41mg	136	31%

GREEN RICE

2 tablespoons margarine or butter
3 cups cooked brown rice (about 1 cup raw)
½ teaspoon salt
¼ teaspoon pepper
½ cup chopped parsley
½ teaspoon dill (oregano, thyme, or basil may be substituted)
3 tablespoons sliced scallions

Melt margarine in a skillet; add rice and all remaining ingredients. Gently stir to combine, and heat thoroughly over low heat.

Serves 6

NUTRITIVE VALUES PER SERVING:

FAT	FIBER	VIT. A	VIT. C	CAL	CAL FROM FAT
4.63gm	2.80gm	644 IU	9.59mg	153	27%

LEMON RICE

¼ cup fresh lemon juice
1 cup raw brown rice
1¾ cups water
½ teaspoon salt
2 tablespoons chopped fresh parsley

Combine lemon juice with rice, water, and salt in a saucepan. Bring to a boil; stir, cover, and reduce heat to low. Simmer over low heat for 40 minutes until rice is tender and liquid absorbed. Garnish with chopped parsley before serving.

Serves 6

NUTRITIVE VALUES PER SERVING:

FAT	FIBER	VIT. A	VIT. C	CAL	CAL FROM FAT
.72gm	2.25gm	108 IU	6.81mg	114	6%

MAPLE SYRUP OATMEAL

2 eggs, beaten
3½ cups low-fat milk
½ cup maple syrup
2 cups rolled oats
2 tablespoons margarine or butter
1½ teaspoons cinnamon
1½ cups chopped unpeeled apples

Combine eggs, milk, and maple syrup and cook, stirring, for 5 minutes over medium heat. Stir in oats and cook for 5 minutes. Add margarine; remove from heat and stir to melt margarine and combine ingredients. Garnish with cinnamon and chopped apples.

Serves 6

NUTRITIVE VALUES PER SERVING:

FAT	FIBER	VIT. A	VIT. C	CAL	CAL FROM FAT
10.2gm	2.74gm	563 IU	2.91mg	317	29%

PARSLEY-CHEESE NOODLES

½ pound whole-wheat noodles (white may be substituted)

1 cup low-fat cottage cheese

¼ cup low-fat milk

½ cup chopped parsley

¼ teaspoon garlic powder

2 tablespoons melted margarine or butter

¼ cup crumbled feta cheese

½ cup grated carrots

¼ cup finely chopped onion

¼ teaspoon pepper

½ teaspoon salt

2 eggs, well beaten

Paprika

Cook noodles according to package directions and drain. Combine noodles with all remaining ingredients except eggs and paprika. Toss lightly but thoroughly, then stir in beaten eggs. Pour into an 8-cup casserole lightly coated with cooking spray. Sprinkle with paprika and bake, covered, at 350°F for 30 minutes.

Serves 6

NUTRITIVE VALUES PER SERVING:

FAT	FIBER	VIT. A	VIT. C	CAL	CAL FROM FAT
8.57gm	5.41gm	2142 IU	10.1mg	275	28%

PASTA SHELLS WITH PEAS

2 tablespoons olive oil
1 cup chopped onion
1 garlic clove, minced
2 cups chopped tomatoes
2 cups peas, cooked until barely tender
½ pound small whole-wheat pasta shells, cooked
 al dente
1 teaspoon basil
½ teaspoon salt
¼ teaspoon pepper
1 teaspoon sugar
2 tablespoons tomato paste
½ cup water
⅓ cup parmesan cheese, freshly grated

Heat oil; sauté onions until limp. Add garlic and cook 3 minutes longer. Add tomatoes and cook over low heat for 20 minutes.

While tomatoes are simmering, cook peas and pasta, separately, and drain both. Add peas, pasta, basil, salt, pepper, sugar, tomato paste, and ½ cup water to tomato mixture and bring to a boil. Reduce heat and simmer 5 minutes. Sprinkle with parmesan and serve.

Serves 8

NUTRITIVE VALUES PER SERVING:

FAT	FIBER	VIT. A	VIT. C	CAL	CAL FROM FAT
5.12gm	9.1gm	955 IU	25.6mg	212	22%

PASTA WITH GARLIC
AND WATERCRESS

2 tablespoons olive oil
2 cloves garlic, minced
1 scallion, sliced
½ pound whole-wheat fettuccine (white may be
   substituted)
1 cup chopped watercress
½ teaspoon salt
¼ teaspoon pepper

Heat olive oil over medium-low heat. Sauté garlic and scallion in oil for 5 minutes (do not let garlic brown). Cook pasta according to directions and drain. Immediately toss pasta with oil-garlic mixture; add watercress, salt, and pepper, toss again, and serve.

Serves 8

NUTRITIVE VALUES PER SERVING:

FAT	FIBER	VIT. A	VIT. C	CAL	CAL FROM FAT
3.85gm	3.39gm	162 IU	2.58mg	146	24%

PASTA WITH PEPPERS
AND PARMESAN

1 tablespoon margarine or butter
1 tablespoon olive oil
2 red or green bell peppers, quartered and thinly
   sliced
1 clove garlic, minced
½ teaspoon salt
¼ teaspoon pepper
8 ounces whole-wheat fettuccine or other flat
   pasta (white may be substituted)
6 tablespoons freshly grated parmesan cheese

Heat margarine and oil in a large pan; add pepper strips and garlic and sauté over medium-high heat for 5 minutes. Add salt and pepper and cook 2 minutes more. Keep warm until pasta is done.

Cook pasta according to package directions, until al dente. Drain pasta and immediately toss with pepper mixture and parmesan cheese. Serve at once.

Serves 6

NUTRITIVE VALUES PER SERVING:

FAT	FIBER	VIT. A	VIT. C	CAL	CAL FROM FAT
6.41gm	3.87gm	269 IU	48.0mg	220	26%

PILAF

Pilaf is a good side dish to serve when the rest of your menu requires last-minute attention—it cooks off-heat by itself.

2 tablespoons margarine or butter
½ cup sliced scallions
1½ cups bulgur (cracked wheat)
3 cups chicken broth
¼ teaspoon pepper
½ cup chopped fresh parsley

Melt margarine in a large skillet. Add scallions and cook over medium heat until wilted. Stir in bulgur, broth, and pepper and bring to a boil. Turn off heat, cover, and let stand for 45 minutes without removing from burner. Do not remove cover during this time.

At the end of 45 minutes, toss pilaf gently with a fork to fluff and heat gently over low heat until heated through. Sprinkle with parsley and serve.

Serves 6

NUTRITIVE VALUES PER SERVING:

FAT	FIBER	VIT. A	VIT. C	CAL	CAL FROM FAT
5.05gm	4.72gm	768 IU	11.3mg	200	23%

RICE WITH MUSHROOMS

½ ounce dried mushrooms (Italian Porcini are
  recommended)
¼ cup white wine
3 cups chicken broth
2 tablespoons margarine or butter
2 scallions, sliced
1½ cups white rice
½ cup freshly grated parmesan cheese
1 cup chopped fresh parsley

Soak mushrooms in wine for ½ hour, then drain and chop,
discarding liquid. Bring broth to a boil; reduce heat and keep
broth at a low simmer. Melt margarine; sauté scallions in
margarine for 5 minutes. Add rice, stir well, and cook until rice
is golden. Add drained, chopped mushrooms and stir to combine.
  Stir a cup of simmering broth into mushroom-rice mixture.
Cook over low heat, uncovered, until broth is absorbed, stirring
often to prevent sticking. Add another ½ cup of broth and cook
as above until liquid has been absorbed, continuing to stir often.
Repeat this procedure until all the broth has been used.
  Garnish with parmesan and parsley and serve.

Serves 8

NUTRITIVE VALUES PER SERVING:

FAT	FIBER	VIT. A	VIT. C	CAL	CAL FROM FAT
4.38gm	1.79gm	912 IU	14.9mg	183	22%

RISOTTO

4 cups chicken broth
1 tablespoon margarine or butter
2 teaspoons olive oil
1 cup brown rice
1 cup chopped onions
1 clove garlic, minced
1 cup sliced fresh mushrooms
⅓ cup freshly grated parmesan cheese

Heat broth to simmering and keep at a low simmer. Heat margarine and oil in a saucepan. Add rice and stir, then add onions, garlic, and mushrooms. Sauté until onions are limp and rice is golden.

Add 1 cup of simmering broth to rice mixture and cook slowly, uncovered, until broth is absorbed, stirring often to prevent sticking. Add 1 cup more broth, and repeat procedure until all the broth has been used and the rice is tender, about 45 minutes to 1 hour.

Sprinkle with parmesan and serve immediately.

Serves 6

NUTRITIVE VALUES PER SERVING:

FAT	FIBER	VIT. A	VIT. C	CAL	CAL FROM FAT
6.27gm	3.14gm	148 IU	3.32mg	187	30%

SPANISH RICE

1 tablespoon corn or safflower oil
1 tablespoon olive oil
1 cup brown rice
¾ cup thinly sliced onion
¾ cup chopped green pepper
¾ cup chopped tomato
½ teaspoon salt
¼ teaspoon pepper

Heat oils; add rice and onion and sauté over low heat for 10 minutes. Stir in green pepper, tomato, salt, and pepper. Add 1½ cups boiling water. Bring rice mixture to a boil, cover, and cook over low heat for 40 minutes without lifting cover. Fluff with a fork and serve.

Serves 6

NUTRITIVE VALUES PER SERVING:

FAT	FIBER	VIT. A	VIT. C	CAL	CAL FROM FAT
5.35gm	3.14gm	364 IU	33.1mg	167	29%

VERMICELLI-RICE PILAF

½ cup whole-wheat vermicelli, broken into small
     pieces (white may be substituted)
¼ cup sliced scallions
2 tablespoons margarine or butter
1 cup brown rice
½ teaspoon oregano
¼ teaspoon celery salt
¼ teaspoon pepper
2½ cups chicken broth

Sauté vermicelli and scallions in margarine for 5 minutes over
medium heat. Add rice, oregano, celery salt, pepper, and broth
and bring to a boil. Cover, reduce heat, and simmer for 50
minutes. Fluff with a fork and serve.

Serves 6

NUTRITIVE VALUES PER SERVING:

FAT	FIBER	VIT. A	VIT. C	CAL	CAL FROM FAT
5.10gm	2.28gm	176 IU	.76mg	185	25%

VERMICELLI WITH BROCCOLI

1 bunch fresh broccoli
2 tablespoons margarine or butter
3 scallions, sliced
1 clove garlic, minced
2 tablespoons white wine
½ teaspoon salt
1 teaspoon lemon juice
¾ pound whole-wheat vermicelli
1 tablespoon olive oil
¼ cup freshly grated parmesan cheese

Cut broccoli into florets; peel and slice stems. Steam broccoli florets and stems until tender-crisp, then gently run under cold water and drain. Heat margarine; add scallions and garlic and sauté for 2 minutes. Add wine and cook 5 minutes. Add broccoli, salt, and lemon juice and heat through.

Meanwhile, cook vermicelli and drain well. Place hot, drained pasta into a serving bowl and toss with olive oil. Toss the broccoli mixture with pasta and sprinkle with parmesan. Serve immediately.

Serves 8

NUTRITIVE VALUES PER SERVING:

FAT	FIBER	VIT. A	VIT. C	CAL	CAL FROM FAT
6.20gm	8.47gm	1679 IU	53.5mg	241	23%

WHOLE-WHEAT BISCUITS

½ cup plus 2 tablespoons whole-wheat flour
½ cup plus 2 tablespoons unbleached white flour
½ teaspoon baking powder
⅛ teaspoon baking soda
⅛ teaspoon salt
2 tablespoons margarine or butter
1 egg
⅓ cup low-fat yogurt

Combine the dry ingredients. Cut in the margarine with a fork or pastry blender until crumbly. Beat egg with yogurt. Mix with dry ingredients just until moistened. Drop into 6 muffin cups coated with cooking spray, and bake for 20 minutes in a preheated 450°F oven.

Makes 6 large biscuits

NUTRITIVE VALUES PER BISCUIT:

FAT	FIBER	VIT. A	VIT. C	CAL	CAL FROM FAT
5.24gm	1.58gm	208 IU	.11mg	144	33%

WHOLE-WHEAT BREAD STUFFING

Use to stuff a 5-pound chicken or 6-pound turkey. The stuffing may be made ahead and refrigerated, but don't fill the bird until shortly before cooking to prevent bacteria from developing.

¾ cup chopped onion
¾ cup chopped celery
¼ cup margarine or butter
1½ teaspoons poultry seasonings
½ teaspoon salt
¼ teaspoon pepper
½ cup chopped fresh parsley
5 cups unseasoned whole-wheat bread crumbs
1½ cups chicken (or vegetable) broth

Sauté onion and celery in margarine for 5 minutes. Combine poultry seasoning, salt, pepper, and parsley and add to onion mixture. Cook 5 more minutes. On low heat, add bread crumbs about 1 cup at a time, and toss to thoroughly distribute crumbs and other ingredients evenly. Add broth and toss again. When using as a side dish, bake, covered, at 350°F for 30 minutes.

Serves 8

Nutritive Values per Serving:

FAT	FIBER	VIT. A	VIT. C	CAL	CAL FROM FAT
8.86gm	6.40gm	604 IU	8.76mg	307	26%

WHOLE-WHEAT SCONES

3 tablespoons margarine or butter
2 eggs
2 tablespoons honey
$\frac{1}{3}$ cup water
1 cup whole-wheat flour
1 cup unbleached white flour
1 tablespoon baking powder
$\frac{1}{4}$ teaspoon salt
$\frac{1}{4}$ cup nonfat dry milk

Soften margarine in a processor, or with a fork. Thoroughly mix in eggs, then honey, then water, combining well after each addition.

Combine flour, baking powder, salt, and dry milk in a bowl and add to liquid ingredients. Mix just until blended, then knead a few times on a lightly floured board. Pat into an 8-inch circle and cut into 12 wedges. Place wedges on a baking sheet lightly coated with cooking spray and bake for 12 minutes at 425°F.

Makes 12 scones

NUTRITIVE VALUES PER SCONE:

FAT	FIBER	VIT. A	VIT. C	CAL	CAL FROM FAT
4.05gm	1.27gm	194 IU	.12mg	126	29%

YORKSHIRE PUDDING

Because we add some whole-wheat flour in this recipe, the pudding does not rise in the usual manner. However, the taste is wonderful, and the pudding is cut into squares and served directly from the oven as usual.

5 teaspoons margarine or butter
3 eggs
1½ cups low-fat milk
1 cup unbleached white flour
½ cup whole-wheat flour
½ teaspoon salt
¼ cup strong beef broth

Place margarine in a 9" × 13" pan. Put pan at lowest level in a 450°F oven to melt margarine.

While margarine is melting, make batter. Mix eggs and milk together in a blender or processor. Add flour and salt all at once and continue processing until smooth. When margarine is melted, add beef broth and tilt pan to mix. Immediately pour batter into the hot broth mixture and bake for 30 minutes at 450°F. Serve at once.

Serves 8

NUTRITIVE VALUES PER SERVING:

FAT	FIBER	VIT. A	VIT. C	CAL	CAL FROM FAT
5.64gm	1.18gm	289 IU	.44mg	156	33%

8
Sauces and Salad Dressings

SAUCES

Chili Sauce
Creamy Caper-Mustard Sauce
Creamy Garlic Sauce
Dill Sauce
Ginger Sauce
Honey Mustard
Horseradish Cream
Lemon-Yogurt Sauce
Light White Sauce
Madeira Sauce
Marinara Sauce
Mexican Green Sauce
Mint Sauce
Mushroom Sauce
Piquant Tomato Sauce
Sherry-Vegetable Sauce
Spanish Vegetable Sauce
Spinach Pesto
Sweet and Sour Sauce
Thyme Sauce
Uncooked Tomato Sauce

SALAD DRESSINGS

Blue Cheese Dressing
Buttermilk Dressing (or Dip)
Creamy Mustard Dressing (or Dip)
Creamy Soy Dressing
Creamy Yogurt Dressing
Cucumber Salad Dressing
Dill Dressing
Fruit Salad Dressing
Garlic Dressing
Herb-Studded French Dressing
Lemon Salad Dressing
Raspberry Vinegar
Raspberry Vinegar Dressing
Red Wine Vinaigrette
Sour Cream Dressing
Soy-Sesame Vinaigrette
Tangy French Dressing
Watercress Dressing
Yogurt-Chutney Dressing

Sauces and Salad Dressings

If you are conscientious about following a reduced-fat diet, using only the leanest of meats and fish and removing the skin and fat from poultry, the results will certainly be healthful, but also might leave you wanting something more. Plain meat, skinless chicken, and bare poached fish can all be complemented with additional flavor—herbs and spices. But you needn't stop there. A well-executed sauce offers limitless possibilities for interesting and satisfying entrées, and will also dissipate the feeling that "something is missing" (that "something" being fat).

The sauces in this chapter are designed to replace the fat with flavor, moisture, and general sensory appeal. The food looks as appetizing as it tastes delicious. The right sauce will dress up even the plainest piece of white fish, the loneliest slice of turkey breast, or the sparest slice of lean meat. (See "Cooking Methods" in Chapter 4 for the best ways to prepare lean meats, fish, and poultry to ensure tenderness—even the most savory sauce cannot mask a leathery piece of meat or an overcooked piece of chicken or fish.)

This chapter features three categories of sauces: vegetable sauces, creamy-type sauces (lower in fat than typical cream sauce recipes), and herb/condiment sauces. Some of them do contain small amounts of oil or margarine, but the amounts are only a fraction of the fat found in conventional sauces or the marbling of fatty meats.

In this chapter, nutritive values for calories and grams of fat are based on a *one-tablespoon* serving. In most cases, the vitamin and fiber content were not measurable.

Here are a few suggestions you can follow to ensure that your salad, fish, pasta, etc., is less than 30% calories from fat *after* the dressing or sauces is added:

- Make sure that the food that the dressing or sauce will be added to is by itself less than 30% calories from fat. For example, one cup of whole-wheat pasta noodles is 4% calories from fat, four ounces of a broiled white fish is 14% calories from fat, or your basic salad, composed of 1½ cups spinach greens, ½ carrot, ⅓ cup kidney beans, ⅙ cucumber, 1 tomato, and ½ green onion, will be around 6% calories from fat.
- If the dressing or sauce you are using is *less* than 30% calories from fat, and whatever you are adding it to is less than 30% calories from fat, use as much as you like. The percentage of calories from fat of the food combination will always be less than 30%. This suggestion applies to 15 of the sauces and salad dressings in this chapter.
- If the salad dressing or sauce is *greater* than 30% calories from fat, you will need to refigure the fat percentage for the combination of sauce and food. Add the grams of fat from the sauce (per serving) to the grams of fat from the food (per serving) and multiply by 9 (there are 9 calories per gram of fat), then divide that number by the total amount of calories for that food combination. Multiply the final number by 100 for the percentage of calories from fat.

    For example, add the grams of fat from 1½ tablespoons of Spinach Pesto (6.24) to the grams of fat from one cup of cooked pasta (.7). Take the total (6.94) and multiply by 9. Divide the product (62.5) by the total amount of calories (236) (one cup pasta is 172 calories, 1½ tablespoons Pesto is 64.2 calories). 62.5 ÷ 236 = .26, or 26% calories from fat.

If you add 1½ tablespoons of Tangy French Dressing to the basic salad described above, you'll have a total of 29% calories from fat. If you spoon 2 tablespoons of Creamy Sherry Sauce on 4 ounces of broiled white fish, your total calories from fat will be 25%.

Many of the sauce recipes contain tomatoes as the base ingredient. This luscious, vitamin-C-rich vegetable (technically a fruit) is a part of many culinary cultures. Try to imagine French, Italian, or Mexican cooking without the tomato! A fresh, vine-ripened tomato is our first choice for any recipe using tomatoes. If you don't have your own tomato patch or know a generous friend who does, try a produce market, local fruit stand, or a natural food store for home-grown tomatoes. Almost without exception, the usual supermarket tomatoes are *not* vine-ripened and are virtually tasteless. It's pointless to spend time preparing fresh tomatoes with no taste when a good canned tomato will taste better.

A classic Marinara Sauce (spaghetti sauce) and an Uncooked Tomato Sauce are included in this chapter to use with pasta dishes. Spanish Vegetable Sauce has a base of tomatoes and fresh basil and is a perfect accompaniment for beef, poultry, fish, or pasta. It can also be made ahead and frozen in small containers for fast and simple dinners. (See page 224 for directions on how to peel and seed tomatoes quickly and easily.)

To complement the taste of vegetables like cauliflower, broccoli, carrots, or spinach, serve them with Creamy Mustard Sauce, Dill Sauce, or Thyme Sauce. These sauces contain less fat per tablespoon than butter or margarine.

One of the most versatile sauces in this chapter is Light White Sauce. It is a creamy-type sauce that uses low-fat ricotta cheese, milk, and low-fat yogurt as its base. It has a creamy texture and delicate flavor perfect for vegetables, pasta dishes, or fish. Light White Sauce can be embellished by adding various spices—oregano, thyme, dill, parsley—for different flavor variations. Add some fresh chives and chopped parsley to Light White Sauce and spoon over mashed or baked potatoes instead of drowning them in butter.

If you use one of the heavier sauces that contains oil or margarine—like Mushroom Sauce, Horseradish Cream, Madeira Sauce, or Spinach Pesto—only serve a small amount with any entrée. Too much sauce will overwhelm the taste of the meat, fish, poultry, and you'll be eating too much fat.

Pasta—a favorite food of many people—is high in vitamins, complex carbohydrates, and fiber (using the whole-wheat variety) and low in fat. There are a number of delicious sauces in this chapter for pastas, including Marinara Sauce, Uncooked Tomato Sauce, Spanish Vegetable Sauce, Thyme Sauce, and Spinach

Pesto. For an elegant pasta presentation, put drained pasta (vermicelli or shells) on a large, warmed serving platter. Cover the pasta with Marinara Sauce, then spoon 4 tablespoons of Spinach Pesto or Light White Sauce around the edge of the platter. Garnish with sprigs of watercress or parsley. Lasagna Pinwheels with Two Sauces (see Index) is a tasty version of this dish. It also works well with spaghetti, manicotti, fettucine, and cannelloni.

Sweet and Sour Sauce is excellent with fish dishes, chicken, or as a dip for hors d'oeuvres (see Oriental Meatballs). Mexican Green Sauce or Chili Sauce can perk up the plainest of foods, or accompany any kind of Mexican dish (see Turkey Chili with Garnishes).

Most of the sauces can be made ahead and frozen in small containers for fast dinners or meals for one. It takes only minutes to poach a piece of chicken, steam a fresh vegetable, and defrost one of the sauces to serve over both entrée and vegetable.

This chapter, perhaps more than any other in the book, demonstrates what interesting, varied, and delicious foods are available on a cancer risk–reduction diet.

CHILI SAUCE

Use on Mexican food such as chiles rellenos, burritos, and tacos, to add interest to plain meat or chicken.

2 tablespoons diced mild green chilies (canned)
1 cup tomato sauce
1½ tablespoons finely chopped onion
2 tablespoons red wine vinegar
½ teaspoon ground cumin

Combine all ingredients and simmer for 15 minutes. Serve hot.

Makes about 1⅓ cups

NUTRITIVE VALUES PER TABLESPOON:

FAT	CAL	CAL FROM FAT
.04gm	4.02	8%

CREAMY CAPER-MUSTARD SAUCE

This sauce makes a very special entrée out of plain chicken or fish, as well as being a good sauce for vegetables and leftover meat.

⅔ cup low-fat yogurt
⅔ cup mayonnaise
⅓ cup low-fat milk
1 tablespoon dijon mustard
½ teaspoon salt
½ teaspoon paprika
1 tablespoon capers, drained
1 clove garlic, minced

Combine yogurt and mayonnaise. Whisk in milk, then add remaining ingredients and combine well. Serve chilled or at room temperature with chicken, turkey, or fish.

Makes about 1¾ cups

NUTRITIVE VALUES PER TABLESPOON:

FAT	CAL	CAL FROM FAT
4.26gm	42.3	91%

CREAMY GARLIC SAUCE

Especially good on fish and vegetables.

8 ounces tofu, drained (about ½ package)
1 teaspoon dijon mustard
¼ cup finely chopped fresh parsley
¼ cup finely chopped scallions
2 tablespoons fresh lemon juice
1 tablespoon white wine vinegar
½ teaspoon salt
2 cloves garlic, minced (or 1 clove, for a milder flavor)
1 tablespoon olive oil

Mix all ingredients in a blender until smooth. Store in refrigerator. Serve chilled or heat very gently until hot.

Makes about 1¾ cups

NUTRITIVE VALUES PER TABLESPOON:

FAT	CAL	CAL FROM FAT
.80gm	10.5	69%

DILL SAUCE

For fish, chicken, or vegetables. Very good with Seafood Pâté (see Index).

1 cup low-fat yogurt
½ teaspoon dried dill weed
¼ teaspoon salt
2 tablespoons finely chopped green onions

Combine all ingredients well and store in refrigerator. Serve chilled or at room temperature.

Makes about 1 cup

NUTRITIVE VALUES PER TABLESPOON:

FAT	CAL	CAL FROM FAT
.19gm	8.15	21%

GINGER SAUCE

Ginger Sauce is very good with poultry of any kind. It also makes an interesting dip—try it with Oriental Meatballs (see Index).

1 16-ounce can apricots in juice, undrained
¼ cup cider vinegar
¼ cup sliced green onions
⅛ teaspoon cayenne pepper
⅛ teaspoon ground allspice
¼-½ teaspoon ground ginger, to taste*
⅓ cup corn syrup

Remove pits from apricots. Place apricots and their juice in blender, add remaining ingredients, and process until smooth. Place mixture in a saucepan and bring to a boil; reduce heat and simmer gently for 45 minutes.

Makes about 2¾ cups

---

*Ginger is quite spicy. If you like a milder flavor, start with ¼ teaspoon.

NUTRITIVE VALUES PER TABLESPOON:

FAT	CAL	CAL FROM FAT
.005gm	11.9	0%

HONEY MUSTARD

This honey sauce is a very good accompaniment to both poultry and roast beef.

⅓ cup honey
⅓ cup dijon mustard*

Combine ingredients and let set for a few hours to allow flavors to merge.

Makes about ⅔ cup

---

*With only two ingredients in the sauce, it is very important to use a mustard of good quality.

NUTRITIVE VALUES PER TABLESPOON:

FAT	CAL	CAL FROM FAT
.33gm	36.4	8%

HORSERADISH CREAM

This is wonderful on both beef and baked potatoes. Try it on sandwiches instead of mayonnaise.

¼ **cup mayonnaise**
¼ **cup low-fat yogurt**
1½ **tablespoons fresh lime juice**
1 **tablespoon horseradish**
1½ **teaspoons dijon mustard**
¼ **teaspoon salt**

Combine mayonnaise and yogurt and blend well. Add remaining ingredients and mix to combine. Sauce is best if made a few hours ahead of time, and stored in refrigerator.

Makes about ⅔ cup

NUTRITIVE VALUES PER TABLESPOON:

FAT	CAL	CAL FROM FAT
4.05gm	39.7	92%

LEMON-YOGURT SAUCE

This piquant sauce is good on fish, poultry, and vegetables.

3-4 tablespoons fresh lemon juice
1 cup low-fat yogurt
1 hard-cooked egg, chopped
2 scallions, sliced
¼ cup finely chopped parsley
½ teaspoon salt
¼ teaspoon pepper

Combine all ingredients, using 3 tablespoons of lemon juice, and gently stir to combine. Taste, then add fourth tablespoon of lemon juice if desired. Serve chilled or at room temperature.

Makes about 1¾ cups

NUTRITIVE VALUES PER TABLESPOON:

FAT	CAL	CAL FROM FAT
.32gm	8.8	33%

LIGHT WHITE SAUCE

This sauce has a wide variety of uses, and is a wonderful base for other tasty sauces.

1 cup part-skim ricotta cheese
¼ cup low-fat milk
¼ cup low-fat yogurt
¼ teaspoon salt

Mix all ingredients; refrigerate about 12 hours before using. Heat very gently in double boiler or use at room temperature.

As a second sauce for pasta: bring sauce to room temperature and place a spoonful over each piece of lasagna just before serving—or pour a bit down the length of canelloni or manicotti to make an extra special entrée. Serves 12 when used in this manner.

Makes about 1½ cups

NUTRITIVE VALUES PER TABLESPOON:

FAT	CAL	CAL FROM FAT
.86gm	16.7	46%

VARIATIONS

CREAM SHERRY SAUCE

1 cup Light White Sauce
¼ teaspoon tarragon
1 tablespoon sherry
¼ teaspoon salt
⅛ teaspoon white pepper
2 tablespoons parmesan cheese

Combine all ingredients, and heat very gently in double boiler. Serve with poultry or fish. Makes about 1¼ cups sauce; serves 6.

NUTRITIVE VALUES PER TABLESPOON:

FAT	CAL	CAL FROM FAT
1.55gm	30.7	46%

CHEESE SALAD DRESSING

1 cup Light White Sauce
2 tablespoons red wine vinegar
1 clove garlic, minced
¼ teaspoon salt
⅛ teaspoon pepper
½ teaspoon oregano

Combine all ingredients, and refrigerate a few hours to allow flavors to blend. Will keep in refrigerator for 2 days. Makes about 1 cup salad dressing; serves 10.

NUTRITIVE VALUES PER TABLESPOON:

FAT	CAL	CAL FROM FAT
1.40gm	27.7	46%

MADEIRA SAUCE

This is an elegant sauce with poultry or any type of roast, and enhances both vegetables and potatoes.

¼ cup margarine or butter
¼ cup sliced scallions
3 cups chicken broth
¾ cup madeira wine
2 tablespoons cornstarch
4 tablespoons cold water

Melt margarine in a saucepan; sauté scallions for 5 minutes over medium heat. Add broth and bring to a boil. Add madeira wine, stir to combine, and boil, uncovered, for 10 minutes. Combine cornstarch and water and add to the boiling sauce; reduce heat and simmer until thickened. Serve hot.

Makes about 4¼ cups

NUTRITIVE VALUES PER TABLESPOON:

FAT	CAL	CAL FROM FAT
6.97gm	10.6	59%

MARINARA SAUCE

Marinara is a delicious meatless tomato sauce good with any type of pasta.

1 tablespoon olive oil
2 garlic cloves
½ cup chopped onions
1 14½-ounce can italian-style tomatoes, undrained
1 15-ounce can tomato sauce
1 6-ounce can tomato paste
½ cup red wine
1½ teaspoons basil
¼ teaspoon ground oregano
1 bay leaf
¼ teaspoon salt
¼ teaspoon pepper
1½ teaspoon sugar

Heat olive oil in a large saucepan. Sauté garlic and onions in olive oil until onions are transparent. Puree tomatoes in blender and add to onion mixture. Add remaining ingredients and simmer, uncovered, for 1 hour. Serve hot.

Makes about 5½ cups

NUTRITIVE VALUES PER TABLESPOON:

FAT	CAL	CAL FROM FAT
.19gm	7.2	24%

MEXICAN GREEN SAUCE

Use this sauce to pour over plain chicken or meat, or on Mexican food such as chiles rellenos, burritos, or enchiladas.

3 4-ounce cans diced mild green chilies
1½ cups chicken broth
10 large leaves romaine lettuce
1 teaspoon sugar
½ teaspoon ground cumin
½ teaspoon ground coriander
⅓ cup corn or safflower oil

Puree all ingredients except oil in a blender until smooth. Heat oil in a large skillet and add mixture from blender. Simmer uncovered, 5 minutes, or until thickened. Serve hot.

Makes about 4½ cups

NUTRITIVE VALUES PER TABLESPOON:

FAT	CAL	CAL FROM FAT
.80gm	8.82	81%

MINT SAUCE

Serve Mint Sauce with lamb roast or roast chicken. It is also wonderful served with any spinach dish.

1 tablespoon dried mint
1 cup low-fat yogurt
3 tablespoons fresh lemon juice
½ teaspoon salt
1 clove garlic, minced
½ teaspoon basil
⅛ teaspoon sugar

Combine all ingredients and heat very slowly in a double boiler. Serve hot.

Makes about 1¼ cups

NUTRITIVE VALUES PER TABLESPOON:

FAT	CAL	CAL FROM FAT
.10gm	4.7	20%

MUSHROOM SAUCE

Mushroom Sauce is delicious with any poultry or meat. Spoon a bit on your potatoes or vegetables as well, and you won't need margarine or butter.

3 tablespoons margarine or butter
¼ cup sliced scallions
½ pound fresh mushrooms, sliced
¼ teaspoon salt (or none, if using canned broth)
¼ teaspoon pepper
⅓ cup dry white wine
1 cup chicken broth

Melt margarine in a saucepan; and sauté scallions, mushrooms, salt, and pepper for 5 minutes. Add wine and broth and bring to a boil. Cook over high heat for a few minutes, until thickened a bit. Transfer mixture to a blender and blend all ingredients until smooth. Reheat, if necessary, and serve hot.

NUTRITIVE VALUES PER TABLESPOON:

FAT	CAL	CAL FROM FAT
.91gm	10.9	75%

PIQUANT TOMATO SAUCE

Serve this versatile sauce on plain meats, poultry, and fish, or on pasta or vegetables.

2 tablespoons margarine or butter
1 cup chopped onions
1 clove garlic, minced
2 cups peeled, seeded, and chopped fresh tomatoes (to peel and seed, see page 224)
1-2 tablespoons horseradish
¼ teaspoon sugar
¼ teaspoon salt
¼ teaspoon pepper
½ teaspoon thyme

Melt margarine over medium heat and sauté onions and garlic until onions are transparent. Add tomatoes, 1 tablespoon horseradish, sugar, salt, pepper, and thyme. Taste, and add the second tablespoon of horseradish, if desired.

Bring to a boil; reduce heat and simmer, covered, for 20 minutes. Transfer mixture to a blender and process until fairly smooth—some texture is desirable. Reheat, if necessary, and serve hot.

Makes about 3¼ cups

NUTRITIVE VALUES PER TABLESPOON:

FAT	CAL	CAL FROM FAT
.24gm	4.6	47%

SHERRY-VEGETABLE SAUCE

Use to enhance meat, poultry, or pasta—a wonderful way to dress up leftovers.

2 carrots, chopped
2 stalks celery, chopped
¼ cup chopped onion
½ teaspoon thyme
¼ teaspoon salt
¼ teaspoon pepper
1¼ cups sherry
2 cups chicken broth
2 tablespoons margarine or butter, softened
2 tablespoons unbleached white flour

Combine all ingredients except margarine and flour and bring to a boil. Cook for 30 minutes at a low boil, uncovered. Transfer sauce to blender and puree; return to saucepan. Bring to a boil again. Mix margarine and flour together, and whisk into sauce; combine well. Simmer, uncovered, for 5 minutes to thicken. Serve hot. This sauce freezes well.

Makes about 5¼ cups

NUTRITIVE VALUES PER TABLESPOON:

FAT	CAL	CAL FROM FAT
.30gm	8.2	33%

SPANISH VEGETABLE SAUCE

Use Spanish Vegetable Sauce on poultry, meat, fish, or pasta. It is also distinctive with vegetables or on baked potatoes.

12 large ripe tomatoes, peeled, seeded, and choppped (to peel and seed, see page 224)
2 green bell peppers, seeded and chopped
2 onions, chopped
2 carrots, chopped
6 celery stalks, chopped
¼ cup chopped chives
¼ cup chopped fresh parsley
¼ cup chopped fresh basil (or 1 teaspoon dried basil)
3 cloves garlic, minced
1 6-ounce can tomato paste
½ teaspoon sugar

Combine all ingredients and puree—in batches—in blender or food processor until fairly smooth, leaving some texture. Transfer to a saucepan and simmer, uncovered, for 45 minutes. This sauce freezes well.

Makes about 12½ cups

NUTRITIVE VALUES PER TABLESPOON:

FAT	CAL	CAL FROM FAT
.02	3.0	7%

SPINACH PESTO

Try this wonderful sauce on chicken or fish.

2 cups chopped fresh spinach leaves (2 ounces)
1 cup chopped fresh basil leaves (1 ounce)
2 cloves garlic, minced
½ cup parmesan cheese, freshly grated
⅓ cup olive oil
¼ teaspoon salt
¼ teaspoon dried basil

Blend all ingredients in blender or food processor; transfer to saucepan and heat over very low heat. Serve hot.

If serving on pasta, boil ½ pound of pasta and top with the sauce—serves 6 as a side dish. Ordinarily, ½ pound of pasta serves 4; however, because this recipe is higher in fat than most, we suggest this smaller portion.

Makes about 1¼ cups

NUTRITIVE VALUES PER TABLESPOON:

FAT	CAL	CAL FROM FAT
4.16gm	42.8	88%

SWEET AND SOUR SAUCE

2 tablespoons corn or safflower oil
1 medium green bell pepper, chopped
1 medium onion, chopped
1 15-ounce can pineapple chunks in juice, undrained
⅓ cup sugar
¼ cup white vinegar
1 teaspoon soy sauce
¼ cup catsup
2 tablespoons cornstarch
2 tablespoons water

Heat oil in a large skillet; sauté bell pepper and onion in oil for 5 minutes. Add all remaining ingredients except cornstarch and water and simmer 10 minutes. Mix cornstarch and water, add to sauce, and bring to a boil. Simmer, stirring constantly, until thickened. Serve hot.

If using as a dip for small meatballs or hors d'oeuvres, puree in blender to a smoother texture.

Makes about 4½ cups

NUTRITIVE VALUES PER TABLESPOON:

FAT	CAL	CAL FROM FAT
.40gm	12.4	29%

THYME SAUCE

4 tablespoons margarine or butter
2 tablespoons minced onion
½ teaspoon thyme
½ teaspoon salt
¼ teaspoon pepper
2 tablespoons unbleached white flour
1½ cups low-fat milk
¼ cup chopped fresh parley

Melt margarine. Add onion, thyme, salt, and pepper and sauté 5 minutes. Add flour and blend. Add milk and bring to a boil; reduce heat and whisk until smooth and thickened. Add parsley and serve hot. Serve with fish, poultry, or vegetables.

Makes about 2 cups

NUTRITIVE VALUES PER TABLESPOON:

FAT	CAL	CAL FROM FAT
1.66gm	20.5	73%

UNCOOKED TOMATO SAUCE

Good on vegetables or with pasta—it makes enough sauce for ½ pound of pasta, which serves 8 as a side dish.

2 pounds ripe tomatoes, peeled seeded, and chopped (to peel and seed, see page 224)
½ cup onions, finely chopped
1 large clove garlic, minced
¼ cup chopped fresh basil (or 1 teaspoon dried)
¼ cup chopped fresh parsley
⅓ cup olive oil
¾ teaspoon salt
½ teaspoon pepper

Mix all ingredients; let set at least 1 hour before serving. May be heated or served at room temperature.

Makes about 4¼ cups

NUTRITIVE VALUES PER TABLESPOON:

FAT	CAL	CAL FROM FAT
1.09gm	12.5	79%

SALAD DRESSINGS

Any salad is incomplete without the right dressing. On a well-planned, reduced-fat diet, salad dressings should be as low in fat as possible. But they should also taste delicious—otherwise there is no point in even serving a salad. Forget any prejudices you might have against low-fat or fat-free dressings. The dressings in this chapter are satisfying and savory, but still conform to the dietary guidelines of reduced fat. (Be sure to stick to the portion size!)

Oil-based dressings are probably the most popular and versatile. All the classic vinaigrettes begin with a little oil (and vinegar or lemon juice). In our recipes, we suggest olive oil, or corn or safflower oil, or a combination of these for vinaigrette dressings.

Corn, safflower, sunflower, and soy, are all *polyunsaturated* oils (oils with two or more double bonds in their carbon chain structure). Serum cholesterol levels can be lowered—reducing the risk of heart disease—by substituting some of the saturated fats (no double bonds) in our diet with polyunsaturated oils. Some recent studies suggest that monounsaturated fats (one double bond) may also be helpful toward lowering the risk of heart disease. Olive oil is a monounsaturated oil.

If you like to use olive oil and are a cost-conscious consumer, Spanish olive oil (including the "virgin" variety) is cheaper than Italian olive oil and has a richer bouquet and taste. Whether you use Italian or Spanish, "virgin" olive oil tastes better than "pure" olive oil. It costs a little more, but it is worth it.

If you don't care for olive oil, safflower oil is so light that it will not affect the taste of the condiments in the dressing. Sometimes corn or vegetable oil has a rather heavy flavor.

Because oil is 100% calories from fat, we have halved the amounts of oil by adding vegetable or chicken broth to these dressings. The mixture of oil and broth gives the dressings the desired taste and texture with half the amount of fat. You will need less dressing in general if the salad is perfectly dry before tossing. Any water left on salad greens will dilute the dressing, which dilutes the taste. Another effective way of cutting down on the amount of dressing you use is to toss the salad in a bowl much larger than needed. This makes it easy to coat the salad evenly and you won't find any wasted dressing at the bottom of the bowl. (You also don't end up with lettuce leaves or cherry tomatoes on the floor.)

Low-fat yogurt and buttermilk are wonderful bases for creamy-type dressings and add only a small amount of dietary fat. They both have a creamy texture and blend well with herbs and spices for delicious salad dressings and dips. In some dressing recipes, low-fat yogurt or buttermilk is combined with a small amount of mayonnaise. This adds to the creaminess of the texture and gives the dressing a richer taste. Be sure to use real mayonnaise, not "salad dressing"—otherwise, the taste will be too strong. Creamy Mustard Dressing, Buttermilk Dressing, and Blue Cheese Dressing are all tasty versions of creamy salad dressings.

You will find that many dressings in this chapter are suitable for any type of salad, from small dinner salads to hearty full-meal salads. Don't forget about the dressings in Chapter 3—like Spinach Salad Supreme Dressing and the dressing for Black-eyed Peas Vinaigrette. Added to the variety of dressings in this chapter, your salad possibilities are endless.

Savor your salad course—knowing that the dressings are just right for a cancer risk–reduction diet and still taste delicious.

BLUE CHEESE DRESSING

This dressing may also be used as a dip.

½ cup low-fat yogurt
¼ cup crumbled blue cheese
1 tablespoon white wine vinegar
2 tablespoons olive oil
¼ teaspoon white pepper
1 clove garlic, minced

Mix all ingredients together in blender and refrigerate.

Makes about 1 cup

NUTRITIVE VALUES PER TABLESPOON:

FAT	CAL	CAL FROM FAT
2.56gm	28.99	80%

BUTTERMILK DRESSING (OR DIP*)

¼ cup buttermilk
2 tablespoons low-fat yogurt
2 tablespoons mayonnaise
1 tablespoon corn or safflower oil
1 small clove garlic, minced
¼ teaspoon salt
2 tablespoons finely chopped parsley
½ teaspoon oregano

Blend all ingredients together. Flavor is enhanced if dressing is made a few hours ahead and refrigerated until serving time.

Makes about ⅔ cup

---

*To use as a dip, add 2 tablespoons buttermilk instead of ¼ cup buttermilk.

NUTRITIVE VALUES PER TABLESPOON:

FAT	CAL	CAL FROM FAT
3.34gm	33.2	91%

CREAMY MUSTARD DRESSING (OR DIP*)

Makes a wonderful dip for artichokes, asparagus, or broccoli.

⅓ cup low-fat yogurt
⅓ cup mayonnaise
⅓ cup low-fat milk
1 teaspoon dijon mustard
½ teaspoon tarragon
¼ teaspoon salt

Blend all ingredients; refrigerate for several hours before serving.

Makes about 1 cup dressing, or ⅔ cup dip

---

*To use as a dip, add 1 teaspoon drained, chopped capers and omit milk.

NUTRITIVE VALUES PER TABLESPOON:

FAT	CAL	CAL FROM FAT
3.76gm	37.9	89%

CREAMY SOY DRESSING

This is wonderful on spinach salad.

¼ cup mayonnaise
½ cup low-fat yogurt
2 tablespoons soy sauce
1 tablespoon orange juice

Combine all ingredients in blender until smooth. Store in refrigerator. For an "Oriental" salad, use Creamy Soy Dressing with lettuce, mandarin oranges, and sliced green bell pepper.

Makes about 1 cup

NUTRITIVE VALUES PER TABLESPOON:

FAT	CAL	CAL FROM FAT
3.01gm	31.3	87%

CREAMY YOGURT DRESSING

1 tablespoon olive oil
½ cup low-fat yogurt
1½ teaspoons white wine vinegar
¼ teaspoon paprika
¼ teaspoon salt
¼ teaspoon oregano
⅛ teaspoon pepper

Mix all ingredients well and allow to set for at least 1 hour to develop flavors. Store in refrigerator.

Makes about ⅔ cup

NUTRITIVE VALUES PER TABLESPOON:

FAT	CAL	CAL FROM FAT
1.52gm	19.2	71%

CUCUMBER SALAD DRESSING

This is also a refreshing dressing for chilled poached salmon or chicken.

1 medium cucumber
1 tablespoon chopped scallions
2 teaspoons red wine vinegar
½ cup low-fat yogurt
¼ teaspoon sugar
½ teaspoon salt
⅛ teaspoon pepper
1 clove garlic, minced

Peel cucumber and cut in half, lengthwise. Scoop out seeds and grate cucumber. Squeeze out excess liquid. Combine remaining ingredients with grated cucumber, and store in refrigerator.

Makes about 1⅓ cups

NUTRITIVE VALUES PER TABLESPOON:

FAT	CAL	CAL FROM FAT
.08gm	4.1	18%

DILL DRESSING

Dill Dressing also makes a nice, light sauce for chilled salmon or leftover chicken.

½ cup low-fat yogurt
½ teaspoon dried dill weed
½ teaspoon salt
¼ teaspoon pepper
1 tablespoon red wine vinegar

Combine all ingredients and allow flavors to blend for at least 1 hour. Store in refrigerator.

Makes about ½ cup

NUTRITIVE VALUES PER TABLESPOON:

FAT	CAL	CAL FROM FAT
.19gm	8.2	21%

FRUIT SALAD DRESSING

This is an excellent dressing for a fruit salad or an arrangement of fruits.

¾ cup low-fat yogurt
1 tablespoon honey
¼ cup orange juice
½ teaspoon dried mint

Mix all ingredients in blender until smooth. Store in refrigerator.

Makes about 1 cup

NUTRITIVE VALUES PER TABLESPOON:

FAT	CAL	CAL FROM FAT
.16gm	11.7	12%

GARLIC DRESSING

½ cup olive oil
½ cup vegetable or chicken broth
¼ cup white wine vinegar
2 tablespoons lemon juice
3 cloves garlic, minced
1 teaspoon dijon mustard
½ teaspoon sugar
½ teaspoon salt
¼ teaspoon pepper

Combine all ingredients in blender and mix well.

Makes about 1½ cups

NUTRITIVE VALUES PER TABLESPOON:

FAT	CAL	CAL FROM FAT
4.71gm	42.6	99%

HERB-STUDDED FRENCH DRESSING

This flavorful dressing is very light and refreshing.

¼ cup olive oil
⅔ cup chicken or vegetable broth
2 medium garlic cloves, minced
½ teaspoon tarragon
½ teaspoon basil
½ teaspoon thyme
2 tablespoons white wine vinegar
2 tablespoons fresh lemon juice
¼ teaspoon salt
¼ teaspoon pepper
¼ cup chopped fresh parsley

Combine all ingredients; mix well in blender.

Makes about 1⅓ cups

NUTRITIVE VALUES PER TABLESPOON:

FAT	CAL	CAL FROM FAT
2.74gm	25.35	97%

LEMON SALAD DRESSING

We always recommend fresh lemon juice, but in Lemon Salad dressing it is essential. This dressing is wonderful on spinach salad.

¼ cup olive oil
¼ cup vegetable or chicken broth
¼ cup fresh lemon juice
¼ teaspoon salt
¼ teaspoon white pepper
1 clove garlic, minced
½ teaspoon basil

Mix all ingredients well in blender.

Makes about ¾ cup

NUTRITIVE VALUES PER TABLESPOON:

FAT	CAL	CAL FROM FAT
4.54gm	41.6	98%

RASPBERRY VINEGAR

Raspberry vinegar can be purchased, but we suggest making it—it is less expensive and just as tasty. Note that the vinegar needs to "develop" in the refrigerator for 3 weeks before straining and using.

1 pound raspberries, fresh, or frozen without sugar

1 cup sugar

4 cups good quality red or white wine vinegar (white will produce a somewhat more delicate flavor)

In a *nonmetallic* pan, simmer all ingredients slowly for 10 minutes. Refrigerate, covered, in a *nonmetallic* container for 3 weeks. Strain through a mesh sieve, pressing pulp to extract juice from berries. Store in refrigerator.

USES

As a vinegar in salad dressings.

As a low-calorie salad dressing just by itself.

As a sauce: Mix equal amounts of Raspberry Vinegar with melted margarine or butter and spoon over chicken or fish—makes a delicious sauce.

As a hostess gift: Give some Raspberry Vinegar in an attractive bottle as a hostess gift, instead of the usual wine or candy.

Makes about 7 cups

NUTRITIVE VALUES PER TABLESPOON:

FAT	CAL	CAL FROM FAT
.005gm	2.36	2%

RASPBERRY VINEGAR DRESSING

Wonderful, using the Raspberry Vinegar from the previous recipe.

2 tablespoons vegetable or chicken broth
6 tablespoons corn or safflower oil
¼ cup raspberry vinegar
½ teaspoon dijon mustard
½ teaspoon salt

Whisk all ingredients together until well combined. Store in refrigerator.

Makes about ¾ cup

NUTRITIVE VALUES PER TABLESPOON:

FAT	CAL	CAL FROM FAT
6.80gm	64.0	96%

RED WINE VINAIGRETTE

¼ cup olive oil
¼ cup vegetable or chicken broth
2 tablespoons red wine vinegar
2 cloves garlic, minced
½ teaspoon oregano
¼ teaspoon salt
¼ teaspoon pepper

Combine all ingredients in blender and process until smooth.

Makes about ⅔ cup

NUTRITIVE VALUES PER TABLESPOON:

FAT	CAL	CAL FROM FAT
5.42gm	48.6	100%

SOUR CREAM DRESSING

⅔ cup low-fat yogurt
⅓ cup low-fat cottage cheese
1 teaspoon fresh lemon juice
¼ teaspoon salt
¼ teaspoon white pepper

Process all ingredients in blender until very smooth. Store in refrigerator.

Makes about 1 cup

NUTRITIVE VALUES PER TABLESPOON:

FAT	CAL	CAL FROM FAT
.23gm	10.1	21%

SOY-SESAME VINAIGRETTE

This is especially tasty on spinach salad, or on a salad with chicken or fish added to make a light meal.

1 teaspoon toasted sesame seeds
¼ cup olive oil
¼ cup vegetable or chicken broth
1 teaspoon dijon mustard
¼ cup fresh lemon juice
¼ teaspoon pepper
1½ teaspoons soy sauce

To toast sesame seeds, heat for 5 minutes in an ungreased frying pan, tossing frequently, until golden brown. Mix all ingredients together; blend well in blender.

Makes about ¾ cup

NUTRITIVE VALUES PER TABLESPOON:

FAT	CAL	CAL FROM FAT
4.34gm	40.2	97%

TANGY FRENCH DRESSING

¼ cup olive oil
¼ cup vegetable or chicken broth
¼ cup white wine vinegar
2 tablespoons catsup
1 teaspoon sugar
¼ teaspoon paprika
½ teaspoon salt
⅛ teaspoon pepper
¼ teaspoon dry mustard

Combine all ingredients in blender and mix well.

Makes about 1 cup

NUTRITIVE VALUES PER TABLESPOON:

FAT	CAL	CAL FROM FAT
3.61gm	36.2	90%

WATERCRESS DRESSING

¼ cup olive oil
1 cup chopped watercress leaves
¼ cup vegetable or chicken broth
1 tablespoon fresh lemon juice
2 tablespoons white wine vinegar
¼ teaspoon salt
½ teaspoon dijon mustard
¼ teaspoon sugar

Combine all ingredients and process well in blender.

Makes about 1½ cups

NUTRITIVE VALUES PER TABLESPOON:

FAT	CAL	CAL FROM FAT
2.18gm	20.0	98%

YOGURT-CHUTNEY DRESSING

This is especially tasty on spinach, fruit, and chicken salads.

1 cup low-fat yogurt
2 tablespoons chopped chutney
½ teaspoon curry powder
2 tablespoons oil

Combine all ingredients in blender until smooth. Store in refrigerator.

Makes about 1¼ cups

NUTRITIVE VALUES PER TABLESPOON:

FAT	CAL	CAL FROM FAT
1.54gm	24.6	56%

9
Desserts

Ambrosia
Amor Polenta
Apple-Brandy Aspic
Apple Crisp
Applesauce Cake
Apricot Cobbler
Apricot Meringues
Apricot Mousse
Baked Apple Souffles
Baked Pancake
Blackberry Cantaloupe
Brandied Fruit Custard
Brandy-Apricot Pears
Cantaloupe Ice
Cherry-Apricot Flan
Cinnamon-Apple Cake
Cinnamon Crunch
Cranberry-Orange Mold
Creamy Vanilla Pudding

Elegant Cantaloupe and Fruit
Ginger Fruit
Gingerbread with Orange Sauce
Glazed Oranges
Granola Balls
Lemon-Lime Snow
Lemon Squares
Mandarin Orange-Rice Pudding
Norwegian Pancakes
Oatmeal Cake
Oatmeal Shortbread
Peanut Butter-Oatmeal Cookies
Pineapple Cake
Pumpkin Bars
Pumpkin Custard Pie
Raspberry-Apricot Cloud
Strawberry Chiffon
Tropical Cantaloupe

Desserts

Dessert, the most whimsical and frivolous course of all, hooks the sweet tooth in all of us. Who can resist ending a meal with a luscious dessert? (Nobody we know, the authors included!) This chapter is dedicated to those of you who immediately scan a restaurant menu for the dessert listings even before you have decided on an entrée.

"Luscious" doesn't have to mean desserts prohibitively laden with fat or sugar. There are an abundance of recipes on a cancer risk–reduction eating plan that are appealing to the eye as well as to an appetite for sweets. Desserts in this chapter are also higher in vitamins and fiber and lower in fat than usual dessert offerings.

Fruits contain a certain amount of natural sugar. Even in their raw state, a juicy orange or a wedge of fresh melon can satisfy the desire for a sweet dessert. But fruit can also be dressed up to yield rich-tasting and elegant desserts.

Cantaloupe, which is loaded with beta-carotene, vitamin C, and a good amount of fiber, is a perfect example. Consider the following variations:

- *Blackberry Cantaloupe:* Heat fresh or frozen blackberries with a bit of sugar, add cornstarch to thicken, and flavor with vanilla and brandy. Place this rich sauce under sliced cantaloupe and garnish with mint leaves. The sweet/tart sauce is a perfect complement to the melon, and the presentation is beautiful—a deep purple swirled under the soft melon color, dotted with bright green mint leaves. It also supplies 5 grams of fiber per serving.

- Blend ripe cantaloupe pieces with egg white, a little sugar, and a bit of fresh lemon juice. Freeze for a few hours, stirring occasionally, and you have Cantaloupe Ice.
- Mix cantaloupe chunks with raspberries and fresh pineapple, and top with a mixture of orange yogurt and a dash of brandy. This makes Elegant Cantaloupe and Fruit.
- Tropical Cantaloupe is made with fresh pineapple, mandarin oranges, and cantaloupe balls mixed with a strawberry yogurt sauce and sprinkled with toasted coconut and sesame seeds. Leftovers are great for a fruit salad breakfast the next morning.

Cherry-Apricot Flan, which uses beta-carotene-rich apricots as the main ingredient, is another tasty fruit dessert. Or make Raspberry-Apricot Cloud as a party dessert using these succulent fruits: fill a large shell of melt-in-your-mouth meringue with apricots and top with a glaze of raspberry sauce.

Other scrumptious fruit desserts are plentiful: Baked Apple Soufflés, Apricot Mousse, Ginger Fruit, Brandy-Apricot Pears, Glazed Oranges, and a great vitamin- and fiber-rich Apricot Cobbler.

If cake is your weakness, you'll find the recipes in this chapter are higher in fiber and lower in fat than most. Cinnamon-Apple Cake is made with tart green apples and a mixture of whole-wheat and unbleached white flour. Cut into squares, it is easy to pack into lunch bags or use as a snack. It is also the perfect stand-in for high-fat commercial cakes at brunch. Lemon Squares, cut into small pieces, is also excellent for snacks. While sampling cake recipes, try Oatmeal Shortbread, Pumpkin Bars, and Amor Polenta.

Pumpkin Custard Pie rivals any other Thanksgiving pie you've eaten. Its oatmeal crust has less fat than a conventional piecrust, contains a good amount of fiber, and is delicious—and its pumpkin custard filling is beta-carotene–rich.

Mouth-watering puddings and custards include Creamy Vanilla Pudding, Strawberry Chiffon, and Apricot Mousse. They are made with low-fat milk and a minimum of margarine, but are as creamy and smooth as any commercial products, and are full of vitamins, too. Apricot Mousse is rich in vitamin A, and Strawberry Chiffon vitamin C.

Children gobble up Granola Balls and Peanut Butter–Oatmeal Cookies, two great lunch box favorites, and feast on Lemon-Lime Snow, Apricot Meringues, and Gingerbread with Orange Sauce.

Mandarin Orange–Rice Pudding is a wonderful party variety of rice pudding. The creamy texture of the pudding is accented by bursts of flavor from pineapple, raisins, and mandarin oranges. And Apple-Brandy Aspic and Cranberry-Orange Mold are both perfect buffet dishes for holiday meals.

We hope this rich variety of full-flavored desserts has convinced all of you lovers of sweets that it is possible to have desserts that are both good-tasting and healthy on a cancer risk–reduction diet.

AMBROSIA

2 tablespoons sesame seeds, toasted

½ cup low-fat yogurt

¼ cup honey

2 oranges, peeled and cut into bite-sized pieces

2 bananas, peeled and sliced

1 cup seedless grapes, cut in half

2 unpeeled green apples, cut into bite-sized
    pieces

To toast sesame seeds, heat in an ungreased frying pan for 5 minutes, shaking pan frequently, until golden brown (this releases their flavor).

Mix yogurt and honey together to make dressing. Gently toss fruit and dressing together. Sprinkle with toasted sesame seeds just before serving.

Serves 4

NUTRITIVE VALUES PER SERVING:

FAT	FIBER	VIT. A	VIT. C	CAL	CAL FROM FAT
3.56gm	6.47gm	267 IU	48.6mg	261	12%

AMOR POLENTA

This traditional Italian cake is served with fresh strawberries.

5 tablespoons margarine or butter, softened
1 cup sifted confectioners' sugar
1 teaspoon vanilla
2 whole eggs
1¼ cups unbleached white flour
⅓ cup yellow cornmeal
3 cups fresh strawberries, sliced

Cream margarine and sugar until light and fluffy. Add vanilla and beat again. Add eggs, one at a time, and mix thoroughly after each addition. Combine flour and cornmeal and add to margarine-sugar mixture. Beat until well-combined. Lightly coat a loaf pan with cooking spray, and lightly flour. Place batter in loaf pan. Bake 1 hour and 15 minutes in a preheated 350°F oven. Let stand a few minutes and turn out of the pan. Top each serving with ¼ cup strawberries.

Serves 12

NUTRITIVE VALUES PER SERVING:

FAT	FIBER	VIT. A	VIT. C	CAL	CAL FROM FAT
5.98gm	1.31gm	266 IU	21.1mg	163	33%

APPLE-BRANDY ASPIC

2 cups water

⅔ cup sugar

1 teaspoon fresh lemon juice

3 pounds medium-sized green cooking apples,
    sliced but not peeled

3 tablespoons brandy

1 teaspoon oil

¼ cup wheat germ

¼ teaspoon slivered orange peel

½ cup low-fat yogurt

1 teaspoon cinnamon

½ teaspoon nutmeg

4 teaspoons brown sugar

Bring 2 cups water to a boil; add sugar and lemon juice and
return to boil. When sugar has dissolved, add apples and simmer
over medium heat for about 20 minutes, stirring often to keep
from burning. The apple slices will become almost transparent.
Gently stir in brandy.

Lightly cover a 4-cup dish or mold with the oil. Fit a piece of
waxed paper into the bottom of the mold, then turn it over so
both sides are coated with oil. Mix wheat germ and orange peel
and sprinkle over the waxed-paper-covered bottom of the mold.
Add apple mixture and chill for several hours.

Mix yogurt with cinnamon, nutmeg, and brown sugar. To
unmold Apple-Brandy Aspic, dip mold briefly in hot water, run a
knife around edge of mold, and reverse aspic onto a serving dish.
Remove waxed paper. Slice into 8 servings and top each with 1
tablespoon of the yogurt mixture.

Serves 8

NUTRITIVE VALUES PER SERVING:

FAT	FIBER	VIT. A	VIT. C	CAL	CAL FROM FAT
1.64gm	5.34gm	101 IU	10.1mg	204	7%

APPLE CRISP

9 medium-sized green cooking apples, sliced but unpeeled
3 tablespoons lemon juice
1½ cup rolled oats
1 cup brown sugar
¾ cup unbleached white flour
6 tablespoons margarine or butter, melted
1½ teaspoons cinnamon

Preheat oven to 375°F. Toss apples with lemon juice and place in an ungreased 9″ × 13″ pan. Mix remaining ingredients and sprinkle evenly over apples. Bake for 30 minutes at 375°F. Apple Crisp may be served with a spoonful of plain or flavored yogurt.

Serves 12

NUTRITIVE VALUES PER SERVING:

FAT	FIBER	VIT. A	VIT. C	CAL	CAL FROM FAT
6.78gm	4.14gm	296 IU	7.61mg	246	25%

APPLESAUCE CAKE

½ cup wheat germ
1½ cups unbleached white flour
½ cup whole-wheat flour
2 teaspoons cinnamon
1 teaspoon allspice
½ teaspoon ginger
2 teaspoons baking soda
1 cup raisins
¼ cup chopped almonds
¼ cup corn or safflower oil
2 eggs
2 cups sweetened applesauce
⅓ cup honey

Preheat oven to 350°F. Mix wheat germ, flour, spices, and baking soda. Add raisins and nuts. Combine oil, eggs, applesauce, and honey. Add to dry mixture and blend well. Pour into 9″ × 13″ pan sprayed with cooking spray and floured. Bake at 350°F for 30 minutes.

Serves 8

NUTRITIVE VALUES PER SERVING:

FAT	FIBER	VIT. A	VIT. C	CAL	CAL FROM FAT
11.6gm	4.42gm	73.6 IU	1.91mg	380	28%

APRICOT COBBLER

Served with a glass of low-fat milk, Apricot Cobbler becomes an easy but very nutritional breakfast dish.

3 cups fresh apricots, sliced, or one 28-ounce
　　can, drained and sliced (peaches may be
　　substituted)
1½ cups rolled oats
3 tablespoons brown sugar
2 tablespoons wheat germ
1 teaspoon cinnamon
3 tablespoons margarine or butter, melted

Preheat oven to 350°F. Place sliced apricots in an ungreased 9″ ×
13″ pan. Combine remaining ingredients and sprinkle over apricots. Bake for 30 minutes at 350°F.

Serves 6

NUTRITIVE VALUES PER SERVING:

FAT	FIBER	VIT. A	VIT. C	CAL	CAL FROM FAT
7.45gm	3.08gm	2268 IU	7.76mg	197	34%

APRICOT MERINGUES

4 egg whites
⅛ teaspoon salt
½ cup sugar
9 dried apricots, cut into quarters

Beat egg whites and salt until egg whites hold their shape.
Gradually add ¼ cup sugar, beating until egg whites are stiff
(they won't slide when bowl is tilted). Gently fold in remaining
¼ cup sugar. Cover baking pan with parchment paper, or spread
baking pan with a bit of margarine and dust with flour. Drop
batter from a tablespoon onto baking pan. Bake for 1 hour and
45 minutes in an oven preheated to 180–190°F. After 30 minutes
of cooking, place a quartered apricot into the center of each
cookie and continue baking for 1 hour and 15 minutes.

Makes 36 cookies

NUTRITIVE VALUES PER SERVING:

FAT	FIBER	VIT. A	VIT. C	CAL	CAL FROM FAT
0gm	.08gm	127 IU	.22mg	16.6	0%

APRICOT MOUSSE

8 ounces dried apricots

4 tablespoons sugar

1 cup water

1 tablespoon brandy

2 eggs, separated

2 teaspoons vanilla

1 envelope unflavored gelatin

1¼ cups low-fat milk

Place apricots in a saucepan with sugar and water. Bring to a boil; reduce heat and simmer five minutes. Drain apricots, reserving cooking liquid. Puree apricots with brandy, egg yolks, and vanilla. Cool.

Bring cooking liquid to a boil and pour over gelatin. Stir until dissolved. When cooled, put in blender or processor with pureed apricots and milk and blend well. Transfer to a bowl. Whip egg whites and fold gently into apricot mixture, only until blended. Chill in bowl or 6 individual dishes for several hours, or until set.

Serves 6

NUTRITIVE VALUES PER SERVING:

FAT	FIBER	VIT. A	VIT. C	CAL	CAL FROM FAT
3.02gm	1.80gm	2928 IU	5.79mg	177	15%

BAKED APPLE SOUFFLES

6 medium-sized green baking apples
1 egg, separated
⅓ cup sugar
¼ cup low-fat milk
1 tablespoon grated lemon rind
1 tablespoon lemon juice
2 tablespoons margarine or butter, melted and
    cooled

Preheat oven to 350°F. Remove cores from apples, leaving some apple at the bottom to hold filling. Stand apples upright in a pan in which they fit fairly snugly. Add enough water to cover the bottom of the pan. Bake, uncovered, for about 25 minutes at 350°F, until barely soft when pierced gently with a fork.

While apples are cooking, beat egg white until stiff. In another bowl, beat egg yolk slightly. Add sugar, milk, lemon rind, lemon juice, and margarine to egg yolk and mix until blended. Fold in egg white.

Drain off any liquid from the pan of apples. Pour egg mixture into apple cavities. Pour any extra egg mixture over apples. Return apples to oven and bake, uncovered, until tops are set— about 8 minutes. Serve hot or warm.

Serves 6

NUTRITIVE VALUES PER SERVING:

FAT	FIBER	VIT. A	VIT. C	CAL	CAL FROM FAT
5.43gm	4.33gm	295 IU	10.3mg	177	28%

BAKED PANCAKE

2 eggs
1 cup low-fat milk
¾ cup unbleached white flour
¼ cup whole-wheat flour
¼ teaspoon salt
½ teaspoon vanilla
¼ teaspoon baking soda
¼ teaspoon baking powder
1 tablespoon margarine or butter
2 tablespoons confectioners' sugar
2 cups strawberries or other fresh fruit, chopped

Mix all ingredients except margarine, sugar, and fruit in a
blender or food processor. Melt 1 tablespoon margarine in a
round cake pan in a preheated 450°F oven. When the margarine
is melted, spread margarine evenly over bottom and sides of
cake pan and pour in pancake batter. Bake for 15 minutes at
450°F, reduce heat to 350°F, and bake 7 minutes longer or until
golden.

Mix confectioners' sugar with fruit. Top pancake with fruit
mixture and serve immediately.

Serves 4

NUTRITIVE VALUES PER SERVING:

FAT	FIBER	VIT. A	VIT. C	CAL	CAL FROM FAT
7.43gm	3.05gm	393 IU	42.8mg	236	28%

BLACKBERRY CANTALOUPE

12 ounces blackberries (reserve about 18 berries
   for garnish)
¼ cup sugar
2 tablespoons cornstarch
2 tablespoons water
½ teaspoon vanilla
2 teaspoons fresh lemon juice
2 teaspoons brandy or blackberry liqueur
3 cups cantaloupe, cut into slices
Fresh mint sprigs, or washed lemon or camellia
   leaves for garnish

Heat blackberries and sugar to a boil. Mix cornstarch with water
and vanilla and add to blackberry mixture. Cook on medium
heat, stirring constantly, for 10 minutes or until thickened. Cool
and add lemon juice and brandy. Pour blackberry sauce into 6
individual dishes or 1 serving dish. Arrange cantaloupe slices on
top of the sauce, overlapping or in an attractive design. Garnish
with mint sprigs or leaves and fresh berries. Serve chilled.

Serves 6

NUTRITIVE VALUES PER SERVING:

FAT	FIBER	VIT. A	VIT. C	CAL	CAL FROM FAT
.46gm	4.97gm	2183 IU	39.6mg	99	4%

BRANDIED FRUIT CUSTARD

3 eggs
1½ tablespoons honey
3 cups low-fat milk
¾ cup nonfat dry milk
⅛ teaspoon salt
2 teaspoons vanilla
1½ teaspoons brandy
½ teaspoon cinnamon
¼ teaspoon nutmeg
1 diced peach (unpeeled)
1 diced orange

Combine eggs and honey in blender or processor. Add low-fat and dry milk, salt, vanilla, brandy, cinnamon, and nutmeg and process until combined. Stir in diced peach and orange. Pour into an ungreased 9″ × 13″ pan or 8 individual custard cups. Place pan or cups into a larger pan with 1 inch of hot water. Bake for 60 minutes in a preheated 325°F oven.

Serves 8

NUTRITIVE VALUES PER SERVING:

FAT	FIBER	VIT. A	VIT. C	CAL	CAL FROM FAT
3.96gm	.62gm	528 IU	10.6mg	124	29%

BRANDY-APRICOT PEARS

6 medium pears, peeled, or 12 canned pear
halves, drained
1 tablespoon margarine or butter
¼ cup orange juice
¼ cup apricot preserves
2 tablespoons brandy
¼ cup wheat germ
¼ cup brown sugar

If using fresh pears, cut pears in half and remove cores. Slice each pear half into about 4 slices. Spread margarine over a pie plate or 8-inch-square dish. Arrange pear slices in an attractive design in the dish. Mix the orange juice, preserves, and brandy and pour over pears. Mix wheat germ and brown sugar and sprinkle pears with the mixture. Bake for 20 minutes in a preheated 400°F oven, basting halfway through to moisten topping. May be served hot or at room temperature.

Serve 6

Nutritive Values per Serving:

FAT	FIBER	VIT. A	VIT. C	CAL	CAL FROM FAT
2.94gm	4.05gm	133 IU	12.0mg	195	14%

CANTALOUPE ICE

2 cups ripe cantaloupe, cut into cubes
1 egg white
⅓ cup sugar
2 tablespoons fresh lemon juice
Mint leaves
1 cup fresh berries

Put cantaloupe, egg white, sugar, and lemon juice into blender or food processor, and process until smooth. Transfer to a bowl and freeze for about 2 hours, stirring every half hour. After 2 hours, place mixture back in processor and process for about 10 seconds to smooth it. Cover with plastic and return to freezer for a few hours.

Serve in chilled cups with mint leaves and berries as garnishes.

Serves 4

Nutritive Values per Serving:

FAT	FIBER	VIT. A	VIT. C	CAL	CAL FROM FAT
.36gm	3.45gm	2150 IU	38.0mg	112	3%

CHERRY-APRICOT FLAN

This is another dish that is terrific for breakfast or brunch.

1¼ cups low-fat milk

¼ cup sugar

2 eggs

1 tablespoon vanilla

⅛ teaspoon salt

⅔ cup unbleached white flour

2 tablespoons margarine or butter

1 cup fresh cherries, halved and pitted, or 1 cup
    canned cherries, drained

2 cups fresh apricots, cut into pieces the size of
    the halved cherries (drained canned apricots
    may be substituted)

To make the batter, mix all ingredients except margarine and fruit in a blender or food processor. Spread margarine in a pie plate or an 8-cup baking dish. Pour one half of the batter into the dish and place in a 350°F oven for a couple of minutes—just until batter sets. Remove from oven. Spread cherries and apricots over batter. Pour on the remaining batter and bake for 1 hour at 350°F. Serve immediately, hot or warm (flan does not reheat well).

Serves 8

NUTRITIVE VALUES PER SERVING:

FAT	FIBER	VIT. A	VIT. C	CAL	CAL FROM FAT
5.40gm	1.52gm	1311 IU	5.51mg	158	31%

CINNAMON-APPLE CAKE

4 cups unpeeled tart green apples, chopped
2 eggs
¾ cup sugar
¼ cup corn oil or safflower oil
1 cup unbleached white flour
1 cup whole-wheat flour
2 teaspoons baking soda
2 teaspoons cinnamon
¼ teaspoon salt

Preheat oven to 350°F. Mix apples, eggs, sugar, and oil. Add flour, baking soda, cinnamon, and salt and mix gently but well. Spray with cooking spray and then flour a 9" × 13" baking pan. Put cake batter in pan and bake at 350°F for 45 to 50 minutes. Cool a bit and cut into squares.

Serves 8

NUTRITIVE VALUES PER SERVING:

FAT	FIBER	VIT. A	VIT. C	CAL	CAL FROM FAT
8.88gm	4.54gm	111 IU	4.87mg	305	26%

CINNAMON CRUNCH

4 tablespoons margarine or butter
8 cups Chex cereal (2 each of Corn, Wheat,
    Rice, and Bran Chex)
3 tablespoons sugar
1 tablespoon cinnamon

Melt margarine in a large baking pan in a preheated 350°F oven. Add cereals and toss to coat cereals with melted margarine. Combine sugar and cinnamon and sprinkle over cereals. Toss gently but well to evenly coat all the cereal with cinnamon sugar. Bake for 30 minutes at 325°F, gently but thoroughly tossing after 15 minutes. Toss again after removing from oven.

Makes 24 ⅓-cup servings

NUTRITIVE VALUES PER SERVING:

FAT	FIBER	VIT. A	VIT. C	CAL	CAL FROM FAT
2.19gm	1.29gm	100 IU	6.53gm	67.6	29%

CRANBERRY-ORANGE MOLD

4 cups cranberry juice
4 cups orange juice
4 envelopes unflavored gelatin
1 8-ounce container low-fat orange yogurt
    (optional)

Heat 2 cups of either kind of juice to boiling. Add gelatin and stir until dissolved. Mix with remaining 6 cups of juice and pour into an 8- to 10-cup mold or individual dishes. Cool. Unmold by dipping dish briefly in hot water and inverting onto a plate.

Garnish each serving with 2 tablespoons orange yogurt, if desired.

Serves 8

NUTRITIVE VALUES PER SERVING:

FAT	FIBER	VIT. A	VIT. C	CAL	CAL FROM FAT
.62gm	2.25gm	261 IU	120mg	183	3%

CREAMY VANILLA PUDDING

2¾ cups low-fat milk
⅓ cup sugar
¼ cup cornstarch
⅛ teaspoon salt
1 tablespoon margarine or butter
¼ teaspoon nutmeg
1 teaspoon vanilla
1 egg yolk, lightly beaten
⅓ cup raisins or chopped fruit (optional)

Heat milk in medium-sized saucepan. Mix sugar, cornstarch, and salt together and stir slowly into the milk. Bring milk mixture to a boil over medium heat, stirring constantly. Boil for 1 minute. Remove from heat and stir in margarine, nutmeg, and vanilla. Stir some of the hot mixture into the egg yolk and blend well. Whisk egg yolk mixture back into hot mixture in pan. Cover and chill. When partly firm, raisins or fruit may be folded into the pudding.

Serve 4

NUTRITIVE VALUES PER SERVING:

FAT	FIBER	VIT. A	VIT. C	CAL	CAL FROM FAT
7.65gm	1.02gm	540 IU	2.05mg	258	27%

ELEGANT CANTALOUPE AND FRUIT

½ cup low-fat orange yogurt
1 1-pint basket raspberries (about 2 cups)
2 cups fresh pineapple, cut into small cubes
    (pineapple canned in juice may be
    substituted)
2 tablespoons brandy
1 medium cantaloupe
Mint leaves

Gently toss together yogurt, raspberries, pineapple, and brandy. Cut the top quarter off the cantaloupe. Scoop out cantaloupe seeds and fill with fruit and yogurt mixture. Chill for several hours. Slice into eight pieces, lengthwise, giving each person a melon wedge and some fruit. Garnish with mint leaves.

Serves 8

NUTRITIVE VALUES PER SERVING:

FAT	FIBER	VIT. A	VIT. C	CAL	CAL FROM FAT
.60gm	4.12gm	2160 IU	40.7mg	100	5%

GINGER FRUIT

Ginger Fruit is best if marinated for several hours or overnight to allow flavors to develop.

1½ cups fresh peaches, or 1 16-ounce can peaches in juice, drained

1½ cups fresh apricots, or 1 16-ounce can apricots in juice, drained

2 bananas, sliced

1 cup orange juice

2 tablespoons crystalized ginger, chopped

Mint leaves for garnish

Slice peaches and apricots and combine with bananas, orange juice, and ginger. Marinate 12 hours or more. Garnish with mint leaves, if available.

Serves 6

NUTRITIVE VALUES PER SERVING:

FAT	FIBER	VIT. A	VIT. C	CAL	CAL FROM FAT
.46gm	3.50gm	1353 IU	30.7mg	90.2	5%

GINGERBREAD
WITH ORANGE SAUCE

1 cup unbleached white flour
½ cup whole-wheat flour
¼ cup sugar
½ teaspoon baking soda
½ teaspoon baking powder
½ teaspoon salt
1 teaspoon cinnamon
½ teaspoon ginger
½ teaspoon allspice
½ teaspoon nutmeg
¼ cup margarine or butter, melted and cooled
¼ cup pure maple syrup
½ cup low-fat milk
1 egg, well beaten

ORANGE SAUCE

¼ cup sugar
1 tablespoon cornstarch
⅛ teaspoon salt
¾ cup boiling water
½ teaspoon fresh lemon juice
1½ tablespoons fresh orange juice
1 tablespoon margarine or butter

Preheat oven to 350°F. Combine dry ingredients in a large bowl. In a separate bowl, mix margarine, syrup, milk, and egg. Add margarine mixture to dry ingredients and mix until smooth and creamy. Transfer to an 8-inch-square baking pan sprayed with cooking spray, and bake for 25 minutes at 350°F.

To make Orange Sauce, mix sugar, cornstarch, and salt in a saucepan. Place on stove and add boiling water. Bring to a boil and simmer for 10 minutes, stirring occasionally. Add lemon juice, orange juice, and margarine and stir until blended. Serve warm, on gingerbread.

Serves 8

NUTRITIVE VALUES PER SERVING:

FAT	FIBER	VIT. A	VIT. C	CAL	CAL FROM FAT
8.40gm	1.18gm	363 IU	2.04mg	237	32%

GLAZED ORANGES

6 navel oranges
½ cup orange juice
2 tablespoons sugar
2 tablespoons margarine or butter
1 teaspoon fresh lemon juice
2 tablespoons Grand Marnier or brandy
Mint leaves

Slice tops and bottoms off oranges. Cut off skin and most of the white membrane so oranges will look attractive. Pierce oranges all over with a fork to allow marinade to penetrate inside.

In a small pan, combine orange juice, sugar, margarine, lemon juice, and brandy. Bring to a boil; reduce heat and simmer for 10 minutes, skimming off foam with a spoon. Pour orange juice mixture into a small bowl, leaving foamy particles in a pan. Place oranges in a pie plate or similar-sized dish, and pour the glaze over them. Spoon glaze over oranges every 15 minutes for an hour until the oranges are coated with it. Garnish with mint leaves just before serving. May be served at room temperature, or refrigerated and served chilled.

Serves 6

NUTRITIVE VALUES PER SERVING:

FAT	FIBER	VIT. A	VIT. C	CAL	CAL FROM FAT
4.01gm	2.76gm	467 IU	80.4mg	133	27%

GRANOLA BALLS

2 tablespoons corn or safflower oil
½ cup honey
⅔ cup peanut butter
½ cup nonfat dry milk
4 cups rolled oats
1 cup raisins (optional)

Combine oil and honey and blend well. Add peanut butter and mix thoroughly. Add dry milk and combine well with other ingredients. Add oatmeal, one cup at a time, thoroughly mixing after each addition. Add raisins and thoroughly combine. Roll into small balls and store in refrigerator.

Makes 48 balls

NUTRITIVE VALUES PER SERVING:

FAT	FIBER	VIT. A	VIT. C	CAL	CAL FROM FAT
2.88gm	.98gm	23.9 IU	.18mg	76	34%

LEMON-LIME SNOW

1 envelope unflavored gelatin
½ cup sugar
1¼ cups boiling water
1 teaspoon fresh lime peel
¼ cup fresh lemon juice
1 tablespoon fresh lime juice
2 egg whites

Combine gelatin and sugar. Add boiling water and stir until gelatin is dissolved. Stir in lime peel, lemon juice, and lime juice. Chill, stirring occasionally, until mixture is slightly thickened. Transfer to a large bowl and add unbeaten egg whites. Beat at high speed until mixture is light and fluffy and begins to hold its shape. Pour into a 5-cup serving dish and chill until set. (The top layer will be light and fluffy.) Serve from dish.

Serves 6

NUTRITIVE VALUES PER SERVING:

FAT	FIBER	VIT. A	VIT. C	CAL	CAL FROM FAT
0gm	.21gm	2.3 IU	6.08mg	76.8	0

LEMON SQUARES

CRUST

1 cup unbleached white flour
1 cup whole-wheat flour
½ cup sugar
7 tablespoons melted margarine or butter

FILLING

½ cup sugar
¼ cup unbleached white flour
1 teaspoon baking powder
3 eggs, beaten
6 tablespoons fresh lemon juice
1 teaspoon grated lemon peel
1 tablespoon sifted confectioners' sugar

To make crust, mix flour and sugar; add margarine and mix well. Press flat in an ungreased 9″ × 13″ pan. Bake for 20 minutes in a preheated 350°F oven. Remove from oven.

For lemon filling, mix sugar, flour, and baking powder. Add eggs, lemon juice, and lemon peel and mix well. Pour lemon mixture over crust and bake for 25 minutes at 350°F. Remove from oven and sprinkle with confectioners' sugar. Cool slightly before cutting.

Makes 32 squares

NUTRITIVE VALUES PER SQUARE:

FAT	FIBER	VIT. A	VIT. C	CAL	CAL FROM FAT
3.12gm	.507gm	128 IU	1.39mg	83.3	34%

MANDARIN ORANGE-RICE PUDDING

⅓ cup white rice
3 cups low-fat milk
½ teaspoon salt
⅓ cup sugar
1 tablespoon unflavored gelatin
½ cup cold water
1 teaspoon vanilla
¼ cup raisins
2 eggs, beaten
¼ cup sherry
¼ cup orange marmalade
1 small can mandarin oranges, drained (about 11 ounces)
1 cup crushed pineapple, drained

Place rice, milk, salt, and sugar in a saucepan. Cover and bring to a boil. Turn heat to low and cook, covered, for 30 minutes, or until milk is absorbed. Remove from heat. Mix gelatin with cold water and vanilla and immediately stir into rice mixture, mixing well. Add raisins, eggs, sherry. Stir in marmalade, oranges, and pineapple.

Pack tightly in lightly oiled mold. Chill for a few hours and unmold.

Serves 8

NUTRITIVE VALUES PER SERVING:

FAT	FIBER	VIT. A	VIT. C	CAL	CAL FROM FAT
3.32gm	1.28gm	274 IU	6.90mg	206	14%

NORWEGIAN PANCAKES

3 cups buttermilk
2 teaspoons baking soda
1 tablespoon sugar
1 egg, beaten
1 cup whole-wheat flour
1 cup unbleached white flour
⅛ teaspoon salt
3 cups sliced fresh strawberries

Mix all ingredients except strawberries. Heat griddle coated with cooking spray and spoon on batter. Make pancakes in the usual manner, recoating griddle with cooking spray as needed. Serve with fresh strawberries, adding a small amount of syrup if desired.

BLUEBERRY PANCAKES

After spooning batter onto griddle, sprinkle several blueberries on top of each pancake. When underside is done, proceed as usual, turning pancake over and cooking other side.

Serves 6

NUTRITIVE VALUES PER SERVING:

FAT	FIBER	VIT. A	VIT. C	CAL	CAL FROM FAT
2.78gm	4.18gm	104 IU	43.4mg	230	11%

OATMEAL CAKE

1¼ cups boiling water
1 cup rolled oats
4 tablespoons margarine or butter
⅓ cup white sugar
⅓ cup brown sugar
2 eggs, beaten
⅔ cup whole-wheat flour
⅔ cup unbleached white flour
1 teaspoon baking soda
¼ teaspoon salt
1 teaspoon cinnamon
½ teaspoon allspice

Pour boiling water over oats. Add margarine, cover, and let stand for 20 minutes. Add sugars, eggs, flours, soda, salt, cinnamon, and allspice. Mix thoroughly, but don't overmix. Coat a 9″ × 13″ pan with cooking spray. Pour cake batter in pan and bake for 30–35 minutes in a preheated 350°F oven.

Serves 12

NUTRITIVE VALUES PER SERVING:

FAT	FIBER	VIT. A	VIT. C	CAL	CAL FROM FAT
5.33gm	1.30gm	203 IU	.01mg	163	30%

OATMEAL SHORTBREAD

4¼ cups rolled oats
6 tablespoons unbleached white flour
¼ teaspoon salt
7 tablespoons margarine or butter
¾ cup brown sugar
1½ teaspoons vanilla

Combine oats, flour, and salt. Cream margarine and sugar until fluffy. Add vanilla and mix thoroughly. Add margarine mixture to dry ingredients, using your hands to combine well. Press firmly into a 9″ × 13″ pan coated with cooking spray. Bake for 30 minutes in a 350°F oven.

Cool 15 minutes, then cut into 15 pieces. Any crumbs may be saved to sprinkle over fruit or ice milk.

Makes 15 shortbread bars

NUTRITIVE VALUES PER BAR:

FAT	FIBER	VIT. A	VIT. C	CAL	CAL FROM FAT
6.89gm	1.78gm	231 IU	.01mg	192	32%

PEANUT BUTTER-OATMEAL COOKIES

⅓ cup chunky-style peanut butter
½ cup brown sugar
2 tablespoons margarine or butter
1 egg
1 cup rolled oats
¾ cup unbleached white flour
½ cup raisins
½ teaspoon baking soda
½ teaspoon cinnamon
¼ teaspoon salt
2 tablespoons low-fat milk

Beat peanut butter, sugar, and margarine together until smooth. Add egg and combine until well mixed. Combine oats, flour, raisins, baking soda, cinnamon, and salt. Add to peanut butter mixture and beat well; beat in milk.

Drop batter on an ungreased cookie sheet. Bake in a preheated 350°F oven for 15 minutes, or until lightly browned.

Makes 36 medium cookies

NUTRITIVE VALUES PER MEDIUM COOKIE:

FAT	FIBER	VIT. A	VIT. C	CAL	CAL FROM FAT
1.65gm	.42gm	27.2 IU	.06mg	43.5	34%

PINEAPPLE CAKE

2 cups whole-wheat flour
½ cup sugar
2 teaspoons baking soda
¼ teaspoon salt
1 teaspoon cinnamon
¼ cup chopped walnuts
2 eggs, beaten
1 20-ounce can crushed pineapple, packed in
   juice, undrained
1 tablespoon vanilla

Preheat oven to 350°F. Mix together dry ingredients and nuts. Add eggs, pineapple, and vanilla. Lightly coat a 9″ × 13″ pan with cooking spray and lightly flour. Pour batter into a pan and bake for 40 minutes at 350°F.

Serves 12

Nutritive Values per Serving:

FAT	FIBER	VIT. A	VIT. C	CAL	CAL FROM FAT
2.85gm	2.82gm	69.2 IU	4.55mg	157	16%

PUMPKIN BARS

1 cup unbleached white flour
¾ cup whole-wheat flour
¼ cup wheat germ
½ cup nonfat dry milk
1 teaspoon baking soda
2 teaspoons baking powder
½ teaspoon salt
1 teaspoon ground cinnamon
1 teaspoon pumpkin pie spice
2 eggs
7 tablespoons oil
1¼ cups brown sugar
1 16-ounce can pumpkin
1 teaspoon vanilla

Preheat oven to 350°F. Stir together flour, wheat germ, milk, soda, baking powder, salt, cinnamon, and pumpkin pie spice. Beat eggs, oil, sugar, pumpkin, and vanilla with an electric mixer or blender until light and fluffy. Add to dry mixture and thoroughly combine.

Spread batter in a 9″ × 13″ baking pan lightly coated with cooking spray. Bake for 25 minutes at 350°F or until top springs back when lightly touched. Cool slightly before removing from pan. Cut into 48 bars.

Makes 48 bars

NUTRITIVE VALUES PER BAR:

FAT	FIBER	VIT. A	VIT. C	CAL	CAL FROM FAT
2.34gm	:44gm	632 IU	.50mg	64.2	33%

PUMPKIN CUSTARD PIE

CRUST

4 tablespoons melted margarine or butter
1 egg, beaten
2¼ cups rolled oats
6 tablespoons sugar
1½ teaspoons cinnamon

FILLING

2 eggs
1 cup part-skim ricotta cheese
1 16-ounce can pumpkin
½ cup brown sugar
½ teaspoon salt
1½ teaspoons pumpkin pie spice
1 teaspoon vanilla
1 5½-ounce can evaporated milk

TOPPING

¼ cup chopped nuts
¼ cup brown sugar
¼ teaspoon cinnamon

Preheat oven to 350°F. To make crust, melt margarine and cool. Add egg and mix well with margarine. Add oats, sugar, and cinnamon and combine well. Press into 9" × 13" pan lightly coated with cooking spray, and bake for 20 minutes at 350°F. Remove from oven and cool a bit before adding pumpkin filling. Raise oven heat to 375°F.

For filling, beat eggs with cheese, pumpkin, brown sugar, salt, pumpkin pie spice, vanilla, and evaporated milk until well blended. Pour into pie shell and bake for 1 hour and 15 minutes at 375°F. Make the nut topping by combining nuts, ¼ cup brown sugar, and ¼ teaspoon cinnamon. Sprinkle nut topping over pie, and cool slightly before serving.

Serves 10

NUTRITIVE VALUES PER SERVING:

FAT	FIBER	VIT. A	VIT. C	CAL	CAL FROM FAT
11.3gm	2.26gm	3354 IU	2.48mg	305	33%

RASPBERRY-APRICOT CLOUD

Fresh apricots are poached in a sugar syrup. However, the syrup is drained off, so most of this sugar is not consumed.

8 fresh apricots, or 1 28-ounce can apricots in juice, drained (peaches may be substituted)

2 cups water (if using fresh apricots)

⅓ cup sugar (if using fresh apricots)

MERINGUE SHELL

2 egg whites

¼ teaspoon cream of tartar

⅓ cup sugar

RASPBERRY SAUCE

1½ cups fresh raspberries, or 1 10-ounce package frozen, undrained (strawberries may be substituted)

2-4 tablespoons sugar

1 teaspoon vanilla

2 tablespoons cornstarch

2 tablespoons water

If using fresh apricots, cut in half and simmer them for 10 minutes in 2 cups water mixed with ⅓ cup sugar. Drain well (save sugar syrup to use again). Skip this step if using canned apricots.

To make meringue shell, preheat oven to 375°F. Beat egg whites with cream of tartar until foamy. Beat in sugar, 1 tablespoon at a time, until stiff peaks form. Coat a 9-inch pie or cake pan with cooking spray. Spread meringue over bottom and up sides, leaving a flat center area. Place meringue in a 375°F oven and immediately turn off the heat. Leave 6 hours or overnight. Do not open the door at all during these 6 hours or you will release the heat needed to dry the meringue shell. Leave the shell in the pie or cake pan after it is done.

To make raspberry sauce, puree raspberries with 2 to 4 tablespoons sugar (depending on the sweetness of the berries) and vanilla. Mix cornstarch and water together and add to raspberry mixture. Bring to a boil, immediately reduce heat, and cook over a low simmer until thickened—about 10 minutes. Cool.

Just before serving, fill center of meringue shell with apricots and pour raspberry sauce over apricots. The outside white shell surrounding the dark sauce makes a beautiful color contrast, so don't pour the sauce over the edges of the shell. Serve immediately.

Serves 6

NUTRITIVE VALUES PER SERVING:

FAT	FIBER	VIT. A	VIT. C	CAL	CAL FROM FAT
.37gm	3.29gm	1271 IU	12.4mg	124	3%

STRAWBERRY CHIFFON

3 cups fresh strawberries
½ cup part-skim ricotta cheese
½ cup sugar
½ teaspoon vanilla
1 tablespoon brandy
2 envelopes unflavored gelatin
¾ cup water
½ cup nonfat dry milk
½ cup ice water (ice-cold water without ice cubes)
2 tablespoons lemon juice

Puree strawberries in blender or food processor. Add ricotta, sugar, vanilla, and brandy and blend until smooth. Heat gelatin with ¾ cup water in a small saucepan until gelatin is dissolved. Cool a bit. Blend gelatin mixture with ingredients in blender until smooth.

Pour into bowl and chill until mixture mounds on a spoon. Combine dry milk, ice water, and lemon juice and beat with mixer on high speed until stiff peaks form, about 5 minutes. Fold into strawberry mixture. Spoon into a serving dish or individual dishes and chill until firm, about 2 hours.

Serves 6

NUTRITIVE VALUES PER SERVING:

FAT	FIBER	VIT. A	VIT. C	CAL	CAL FROM FAT
1.89gm	2.04gm	244 IU	46.2mg	151	11%

TROPICAL CANTALOUPE

1 tablespoon coconut

1 tablespoon sesame seeds

2 cups cantaloupe, cut into balls or bite-sized
pieces

2 cups fresh pineapple, cut into bite-sized pieces

1 cup mandarin oranges (or other oranges) cut
into bite-sized pieces

8 ounces low-fat strawberry yogurt

Toast coconut and sesame seeds together in a 350°F oven for 10
minutes, stirring frequently. Cool for a few minutes before
using. Combine fruit with yogurt. Just before serving, sprinkle
toasted coconut and sesame seeds over fruit mixture.

Serves 8

NUTRITIVE VALUES PER SERVING:

FAT	FIBER	VIT. A	VIT. C	CAL	CAL FROM FAT
1.42gm	1.49gm	1082 IU	24.0mg	87.7	15%

10
21-Day Menu
Plan

21-Day Menu Plan

Starred * recipes are in the book.
Total number of calories per day ranges between 1,500 and 2,000.

DAY 1
Breakfast

½ cup blackberries
2 Bran Muffins*
8 ounces nonfat milk
Coffee or tea

Lunch

Chicken Chowder*
Spinach and Grapefruit Salad*
2 whole-wheat rolls
Applesauce Cake*
Coffee or tea

Dinner

Chilled Chinese Noodles*
Teriyaki Halibut* (includes rice)
1 cup steamed broccoli

TOTAL CALORIES	GRAMS FIBER	CALORIES FROM FAT
1911	39	21%

DAY 2

Breakfast

Apple Crisp*
8 ounces nonfat milk
Coffee or tea

Lunch

Black-Eyed Peas Vinaigrette*
2 ounces turkey breast slices
2 slices rye bread
2 slices tomato
2 leaves lettuce
1 teaspoon mayonnaise
2 servings Pumpkin Bars*
Coffee or tea

Dinner

Cream of Broccoli Soup*
Summer Salad*
2 servings Manicotti*
1 orange

TOTAL CALORIES	GRAMS FIBER	CALORIES FROM FAT
1506	31	24%

DAY 3
Breakfast

4 ounces fresh orange juice
2 slices Carrot-Zucchini Bread*
8 ounces nonfat milk
Coffee or tea

Lunch

Lamb and Vegetable Soup*
Salade Niçoise*
1 whole-wheat roll
Coffee or tea

Dinner

South American Squash*
Spanish Rice*
Herbed Beans*
Apple-Brandy Aspic*

TOTAL CALORIES	GRAMS FIBER	CALORIES FROM FAT
1865	49.8	24%

DAY 4
Breakfast

Ambrosia*
2 Whole-Wheat Biscuits* with apple butter
8 ounces nonfat milk
Coffee or tea

Lunch

3 ounces canned salmon on 2 slices rye bread
2 slices tomato
2 lettuce leaves
1 slice onion
1 teaspoon mayonnaise
French Potato Salad*
Pineapple juice
Coffee or tea

Dinner

Chinese Watercress and Cabbage Soup*
Mandarin Orange Chicken with Broccoli*
1 cup cooked brown rice
Cherry-Apricot Flan*

TOTAL CALORIES	GRAMS FIBER	CALORIES FROM FAT
1827	31.5	22%

DAY 5
Breakfast

Apple wedges (1 whole apple)
Maple Syrup Oatmeal*
8 ounces nonfat milk
Coffee or tea

Lunch

Vegetable Basil Soup*
1½ servings Pasta Salad with Fresh Tomatoes*
1 whole-wheat roll
Coffee or tea

Dinner

Curried Turkey and Broccoli*
Pilaf*
Glazed Oranges*

TOTAL CALORIES	GRAMS FIBER	CALORIES FROM FAT
1574	41.7	24%

DAY 6
Breakfast

Elegant Cantaloupe and Fruit*
Norwegian Pancakes* with 1 tablespoon maple
    syrup
8 ounces nonfat milk
Coffee or tea

Lunch

Vegetarian Chili Casserole*
2 servings Marinated Carrots*
1 slice Corn Bread*
Coffee or tea

Dinner

2 servings Lobster Tails Italiano* (includes 2
    slices french bread)
1½ servings Vegetable Salad*
Creamy Vanilla Pudding*

TOTAL CALORIES	GRAMS FIBER	CALORIES FROM FAT
1653	36.3	22%

DAY 7
Breakfast

4 ounces orange juice
2 slices Apricot Bread*
8 ounces nonfat milk
Coffee or tea

Lunch

1 cup honeydew melon cubes
Pasta Primavera*
Oatmeal Shortbread*
Coffee or tea

Dinner

French Onion Soup*
Chicken with Mushrooms and Grapes*
Brussels Sprouts and Chestnuts*
1 slice french bread

TOTAL CALORIES	GRAMS FIBER	CALORIES FROM FAT
1835	37.6	27%

DAY 8
Breakfast

4 ounces grapefruit juice
Apple-Oatmeal Cereal*
8 ounces nonfat milk
Coffee or tea

Lunch

Broccoli Quiche*
Whole-Wheat Scones* with 1 teaspoon
    margarine or butter
Ambrosia*
Coffee or tea

Dinner

Spinach Salad Supreme*
Fish Dijon*
Lemon Rice*
Cranberry-Orange Mold*

TOTAL CALORIES	GRAMS FIBER	CALORIES FROM FAT
1635	31.6	17.5%

DAY 9
Breakfast

1 cup apricot halves
1 serving bran-type cereal
8 ounces nonfat milk
Coffee or tea

Lunch

Vegetarian Lasagna*
Winter Vegetable Medley*
Garlic Herb Bread*
Coffee or tea

Dinner

Artichokes with Shrimp Salsa* (6 pieces)
Mexican-Style Beef Stew*
Braised Fresh Tomatoes*
Green Chili Corn Bread*

TOTAL CALORIES	GRAMS FIBER	CALORIES FROM FAT
1759	51	19%

DAY 10

Breakfast

1½ servings Blackberry Cantaloupe*
1 whole-wheat bagel
1 ounce neufchâtel cheese
8 ounces nonfat milk
Coffee or tea

Lunch

Tomato Soup*
2 servings Pasta and Broccoli Salad*
Amor Polenta* with Strawberries
Coffee or tea

Dinner

2 servings Fillet of Sole Braised in Lettuce*
Curried Rice*
Sweet Potato and Carrot Mold*

TOTAL CALORIES	GRAMS FIBER	CALORIES FROM FAT
1634	37	23%

DAY 11
Breakfast

½ grapefruit
2 servings Apricot Cobbler*
8 ounces nonfat milk
Coffee or tea

Lunch

2 servings Mexican Chicken Salad*
Molded Gazpacho Salad*
2 corn tortillas
Coffee or tea

Dinner

Oven-Roasted Lamb with Vegetable Sauce*
Risotto*
Baked Apple Soufflés*

TOTAL CALORIES	GRAMS FIBER	CALORIES FROM FAT
1800	46	25%

DAY 12
Breakfast

1 cup melon cubes (casaba or cantaloupe)
2 slices whole-wheat toast
2 tablespoons apricot preserves
8 ounces nonfat milk
Coffee or tea

Lunch

Lentil Soup*
Stuffed White Potatoes*
Ginger Fruit*
Coffee or tea

Dinner

2 servings Eggplant Parmesan*
Garlic-Sautéed Spinach*
1 slice french bread
Lemon-Lime Snow*

TOTAL CALORIES	GRAMS FIBER	CALORIES FROM FAT
1453	44	17%

DAY 13
Breakfast

Apple wedges (1 whole apple)
2 Bran Muffins*
1 tablespoon strawberry preserves
8 ounces nonfat milk
Coffee or tea

Lunch

Taco Salad*
Carrot-Zucchini Bread*
Glazed Oranges*
Coffee or tea

Dinner

Vermicelli with Broccoli*
Chicken and Sweet Potatoes*
Mandarin Orange–Rice Pudding*

TOTAL CALORIES	GRAMS FIBER	CALORIES FROM FAT
1721	40	19.5%

DAY 14
Breakfast

1 cup honeydew melon cubes
Cornmeal with Honey*
8 ounces nonfat milk
Coffee or tea

Lunch

Lasagna Pinwheels with Two Sauces*
Italian Vegetable Stew*
Amor Polenta*
Coffee or tea

Dinner

Cabbage Soup*
Corned Beef with Vegetables*
1 slice rye bread
Apricot Mousse*

TOTAL CALORIES	GRAMS FIBER	CALORIES FROM FAT
1780	40	15%

DAY 15
Breakfast

Baked Pancake* with fruit
8 ounces nonfat milk
Coffee or tea

Lunch

Marinated Black Bean Salad*
1 serving Italian Sausages*
2 Corn Muffins*
Coffee or tea

Dinner

Spaghetti with Spinach and Mushrooms*
Julienne of Turnips and Carrots*
Garlic Herb Bread*
2 servings Lemon Squares*

TOTAL CALORIES	GRAMS FIBER	CALORIES FROM FAT
1832	41	26%

DAY 16
Breakfast

4 ounces orange juice
2 servings Apple Crisp*
8 ounces nonfat milk
Coffee or tea

Lunch

Cottage Cheese Enchiladas with Green Sauce*
Spanish Rice*
Brandy-Apricot Pears*
Coffee or tea

Dinner

French Beef with Vegetables*
White Beans*
1 whole-wheat roll
Cantaloupe Ice*

TOTAL CALORIES	GRAMS FIBER	CALORIES FROM FAT
1987	50.3	21%

DAY 17
Breakfast

½ grapefruit
Maple Syrup Oatmeal*
8 ounces nonfat milk
Coffee of tea

Lunch

Crab Melt (3 ounces crab mixed with celery and
    scallions)
1 teaspoon mayonnaise
plus ¼ cup grated part-skim mozzarella on
1 large french roll
Brazilian Rice*
Coffee or tea

Dinner

Broccoli and Cauliflower Neapolitan*
Green salad (with ½ cup kidney beans, 2
    radishes, 8 cucumber slices) and
1½ tablespoons Lemon Salad Dressing*
Strawberry Chiffon*

TOTAL CALORIES	GRAMS FIBER	CALORIES FROM FAT
1602	29.2	24%

DAY 18
Breakfast

1 cup blackberries
Norwegian Pancakes*
8 ounces nonfat milk
Coffee or tea

Lunch

Spaghetti Squash and Rice Quiche*
Specially Seasoned Tomatoes*
2 whole-wheat rolls with 1 teaspoon margarine
    or butter
Gingerbread with Orange Sauce*
Coffee or tea

Dinner

2 servings Chicken Fettuccine*
2 servings Carrots in Garlic Sauce*
Brandy-Apricot Pears*

TOTAL CALORIES	GRAMS FIBER	CALORIES FROM FAT
1822	50.7	21%

DAY 19
Breakfast

¾ cup peaches (canned in juice)
1 serving bran-type cereal
8 ounces nonfat milk
Coffee or tea

Lunch

Spinach and Grapefruit Salad*
Broccoli-Noodle Casserole*
1 small french roll
Coffee or tea

Dinner

Portuguese Cabbage Rolls*
Romanian Vegetable Casserole*
Oven French Fries*
Oatmeal Cake*

TOTAL CALORIES	GRAMS FIBER	CALORIES FROM FAT
1495	47.2	20%

DAY 20
Breakfast

Elegant Cantaloupe and Fruit*
1 egg, poached
2 slices whole-wheat toast with 1 teaspoon
    margarine or butter
8 ounces nonfat milk
Coffee or tea

Lunch

Summer Salad*
Chicken Bouillabaisse*
1 Whole-Wheat Scone*
Ambrosia*
Coffee or tea

Dinner

Chili-Cheese Pie*
Green Rice*
Corn Bread*

TOTAL CALORIES	GRAMS FIBER	CALORIES FROM FAT
1655	33.5	27%

DAY 21
Breakfast

4 ounces orange juice
2 servings Apricot Cobbler*
8 ounces nonfat milk
Coffee or tea

Lunch

2 ounces turkey breast
2 slices rye bread
1 lettuce leaf
2 slices tomato
1 teaspoon mayonnaise
2 servings French Potato Salad*
Pumpkin Custard Pie*
Coffee or tea

Dinner

Vegetable Salad*
Potato-Cabbage Casserole*
2 Baking Soda Biscuits*
Tropical Cantaloupe*

TOTAL CALORIES	GRAMS FIBER	CALORIES FROM FAT
1987	37.3	27%

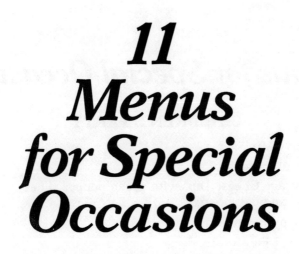

11
Menus
for Special
Occasions

Menus for Special Occasions

CHILDREN'S PARTY

Party Mix*

Tortilla Chips*

Cottage Cheese Dip* with green pepper slices
and carrot sticks

Crispy Parmesan Chicken*

Sweet Potato Fries*

Lettuce with Buttermilk Dressing*, cherry
tomato garnish

Peanut Butter-Oatmeal Cookies*

Lemon-Lime Snow*

ELEGANT DINNER PARTY

Chicken Puffs*

Spinach Dip* served with baguette slices (or
small slices of french bread) and raw
vegetable slices

Seafood Pâté*

Veal Roast Royale* with White Beans*

Julienne of Turnips and Carrots*

Escarole with Raspberry Vinegar Dressing*

Baked Apple Soufflés*

CHRISTMAS BRUNCH

Country Sausages and Potatoes*
Potato-Cheese Pancakes*
Apricot Cobbler*
Whole-Wheat Biscuits* with honey butter
Fresh orange juice

MIDDLE EASTERN PICNIC

Hummus* served with pita bread, red and green
    pepper slices, and cherry tomatoes
Tabbouleh Dip* with romaine lettuce leaves
Stuffed Grape Leaves (Dolmas)*
Lentil Salad with Feta Cheese*
Greek Meatballs*
Cinnamon-Apple Cake*
Cantaloupe balls

ORIENTAL PARTY BUFFET

Chicken Tumble in Lettuce Cups*
Oriental Meatballs*
Foil-Wrapped Chicken*
Chinese Noodle Salad with Peanut Sauce*
Oriental Turkey Salad with Cilantro*
Shredded Chicken Salad*
Steamed carrots marinated in Soy-Sesame
    Vinaigrette*
Sweet and Sour Chicken with Vegetables*
Carrots and Cabbage, Mandarin Style*
Stir-Fried Broccoli*
Chicken Fried Rice*
Mandarin Orange–Rice Pudding*
Ginger Fruit*

THANKSGIVING DINNER

Salmon Spread* with crackers
Mozzarella Vegetable Canapés*
Roast Turkey with Corn Bread Stuffing*
Bourbon-Orange Sweet Potatoes*
Apple-Cranberry Acorn Squash*
Brussels Sprouts and Chestnuts*
Spinach-Filled Tomatoes*
Cranberry-Orange Mold*
Pumpkin Custard Pie*

MEXICAN FIESTA

Refried Bean Platter*, served with Tortilla
  Chips* and carrot sticks
Mexican-Style Beef Stew
Molded Gazpacho Salad*
Mexican Chicken Salad*
Summer Salad*
Spanish Rice*
Marinated Black Bean Salad*
Green Chili Corn Bread*
Green Salsa*
Red Salsa*
Glazed Oranges*
Lemon Squares*

Appendix I
Complete Protein Combinations

You will be eating a "complete protein" when you consume foods in the combinations shown. Where the circles overlap, you have a complete protein if there is a plus (+) sign. In the overlap area with a minus (−) sign, you need to add a food from the legume group to make a complete protein.

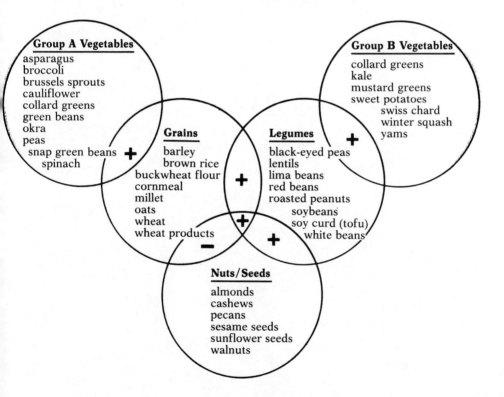

Group A Vegetables
asparagus
broccoli
brussels sprouts
cauliflower
collard greens
green beans
okra
peas
snap green beans
spinach

Grains
barley
brown rice
buckwheat flour
cornmeal
millet
oats
wheat
wheat products

Legumes
black-eyed peas
lentils
lima beans
red beans
roasted peanuts
soybeans
soy curd (tofu)
white beans

Group B Vegetables
collard greens
kale
mustard greens
sweet potatoes
swiss chard
winter squash
yams

Nuts/Seeds
almonds
cashews
pecans
sesame seeds
sunflower seeds
walnuts

Examples:
Combine beans, peas, or lentils with rice
Combine broccoli or cauliflower with whole-wheat pasta
Combine winter squash with lentil soup
Sprinkle sunflower seeds on a salad with kidney beans
Spread peanut butter on whole-grain bread

Appendix II
Nutritive Values (Per Serving)

The following food values were determined by The Food Processor, a computer software program by E.S.H.A. Research.

Cruciferous vegetables are starred * because it is impossible to measure indoles in each one.

FRUIT AND FRUIT JUICES

	Cal from Fat	Grams Fat	Grams Fiber	IU Vit. A	Mg Vit. C	Cal
apple, 1 medium	5%	.50	4.28	74.00	7.80	81.00
applesauce, ½ cup unsweetened	1%	.06	2.56	35.00	1.45	53.00
apricots, fresh, 3 whole	7%	.40	2.23	2769.00	10.60	51.00
apricots, canned in juice, ½ cup	1%	.04	1.75	2098.00	6.10	59.50
apricots, dried, 5 halves	2%	.18	.76	1267.00	2.15	41.50
apricot nectar, 1 cup	1%	.22	1.51	3304.00	36.00	141.00
banana, 1 medium	5%	.55	3.85	92.00	10.30	105.00
blackberries, fresh, 1 cup	7%	.56	10.50	237.00	30.20	74.00
blueberries, fresh, 1 cup	6%	.55	4.93	145.00	19.00	82.00
cherries, fresh, ½ cup	12%	.70	1.60	155.00	5.10	52.00
fruit cocktail, in juice, 1 cup	0%	.03	4.28	757.00	6.80	113.00
grapefruit, ½	3%	.12	1.53	318.00	46.80	37.00
grapes, seedless, ½ cup	7%	.46	1.60	58.50	8.65	57.00
mango slices, 1 cup	4%	.45	2.48	6425.00	45.70	108.00
melon, cantaloupe, 1 cup cubed	8%	.44	1.60	4179.00	54.00	48.00
melon, casaba, 1 cup cubed	3%	.17	1.70	51.00	27.20	45.00
melon, honeydew, 1 cup cubed	3%	.17	1.84	68.00	42.10	60.00
nectarine slices, ½ cup	8%	.32	1.65	508.00	3.70	34.00
orange, 1 medium	2%	.16	2.62	269.00	69.70	62.00
orange juice, fresh, 1 cup	4%	.50	1.69	496.00	124.00	111.00
orange juice, frozen, 1 cup	1%	.14	1.69	194.00	96.90	112.00
orange juice, canned, 1 cup	3%	.36	1.00	437.00	85.70	104.00
papaya slices, 1 cup	3%	.20	1.83	2819.00	86.50	54.00
peach, 1 medium	2%	.08	2.30	465.00	5.70	37.00

peaches, canned in juice, 1 cup	1%	.08	3.60	945.00	8.80	109.00
pear, fresh, 1 medium	6%	.66	3.80	33.00	6.60	98.00
persimmon, 1 large (Japanese variety)	3%	.30	3.00	3640.00	16.50	118.00
pineapple pieces, fresh, 1 cup	8%	.66	2.90	35.00	23.90	77.00
pineapple, canned in juice, ½ cup	1%	.10	2.06	47.50	11.90	75.00
pineapple juice, canned, 1 cup	1%	.20	.75	12.00	26.70	139.00
plum, 1 fresh	10%	.40	2.60	213.00	6.30	36.00
prune juice, 1 cup	0%	.08	3.00	9.00	10.60	181.00
prunes, dried, 5	2%	.22	6.75	835.00	1.40	101.00
raisins, 1 cup	1%	.76	11.20	13.00	5.50	494.00
raspberries, fresh, 1 cup	10%	.68	9.10	160.00	30.80	61.00
strawberries, fresh, 1 cup	11%	.55	3.38	41.00	84.50	45.00
tangerine, 1 fresh	4%	.16	1.60	773.00	25.90	37.00
watermelon pieces, 1 cup	12%	.68	3.20	585.00	15.40	50.00

VEGETABLES

	Cal from Fat	Grams Fat	Grams Fiber	IU Vit. A	Mg Vit. C	Cal
alfalfa sprouts, 1 cup	12%	.13	.67	133.00	4.00	9.66
artichoke, cooked, 1 whole	6%	.20	3.70	180.00	10.00	31.50
artichoke hearts, cooked, 6 oz.	7%	.54	24.00	203.00	8.90	72.00
artichoke hearts, marinated, 6 oz.	72%	13.50	24.00	278.00	51.80	168.00
asparagus, fresh, 1 cup	9%	.30	2.17	1310.00	38.00	29.00
bean sprouts, mung, 1 cup	4%	.20	3.20	20.00	20.00	45.00
beans, black, cooked, ½ cup	4%	.40	9.70	10.00	—	85.00
beans, garbanzo, cooked, ½ cup	16%	4.41	11.00	25.00	—	250.00
beans, great northern, cooked, 1 cup	5%	1.10	15.00	—	—	210.00
beans, green snap, cooked, 1 cup	7%	.25	4.10	680.00	15.00	31.00
beans, kidney, cooked, 1 cup	4%	1.00	19.40	10.00	—	226.00
beans, lima, cooked, ½ cup	2%	.20	5.45	200.00	11.00	106.00
beans, navy, cooked, 1 cup	4%	1.12	15.00	—	—	248.00
beans, pinto, cooked, 1 cup	4%	1.00	18.80	10.00	—	249.00
beans, soy, cooked, 1 cup	39%	10.20	5.20	50.00	—	234.00
beans, yellow wax, cooked, 1 cup	10%	.30	4.10	290.00	16.00	28.00
beet greens, cooked, 1 cup	11%	.37	7.00	8122.00	27.00	30.00
beets, cooked, ½ cup	3%	.10	2.37	15.00	4.90	28.00
broccoli, cooked, 1 cup*	13%	.50	9.40	3880.00	140.00	34.00
brussels sprouts, cooked, 1 cup*	13%	.60	4.50	715.00	135.00	42.00
cabbage, raw, 1 cup*	8%	.15	2.19	106.00	34.40	17.10
cabbage, cooked, 1 cup*	11%	.30	4.05	247.00	48.00	25.50
cabbage, bok choy, cooked, 1 cup*	11%	.30	3.00	5270.00	26.00	24.00
cabbage, red, raw, ½ cup*	6%	.06	1.19	13.00	21.50	9.05
cabbage, savoy, cooked, 1 cup*	—	—	4.96	480.00	45.00	14.40
carrot, raw, 1 medium	5%	.13	3.40	8140.00	4.50	19.50
cauliflower, cooked, ½ cup*	14%	.15	1.20	29.50	34.50	9.75

celery, diced, raw, 1 cup	6%	.10	7.00	304.00	11.00	15.00
chard, Swiss, cooked, 1 cup	11%	.40	6.80	9450.00	28.00	32.00
collard greens, cooked, 1 cup	19%	1.30	7.00	14,820.00	144.00	63.00
corn, yellow, 1 ear	10%	.80	4.00	308.00	7.00	72.00
corn, frozen, ½ cup	7%	.50	4.70	290.00	4.00	65.00
eggplant, cooked, 1 cup	9%	.40	4.50	20.00	6.00	38.00
escarole, 1 cup	4%	.05	.75	1325.00	32.00	12.00
kale greens, cooked, 1 cup*	17%	.80	8.00	9130.00	102.00	43.00
leeks, cooked, ½ cup	11%	.15	1.95	20.00	7.50	12.00
lentils, cooked, ½ cup	4%	.48	4.50	19.00	—	99.00
lettuce, iceburg, 1 cup	21%	.16	.82	180.00	3.70	6.80
lettuce, romaine, 1 cup	19%	.21	.82	1050.00	10.00	10.00
mustard greens, cooked, 1 cup*	17%	.60	7.00	8120.00	67.00	32.00
okra, cooked, ½ cup	10%	.25	2.56	390.00	16.00	23.00
onions, green (scallions), ¼ cup	5%	.05	.78	500.00	8.00	9.00
peas, black-eyed, cooked, 1 cup	7%	1.30	13.00	580.00	28.00	178.00
peas, green, cooked, 1 cup	6%	.60	17.00	860.00	28.00	99.00
pepper, green, raw, ½ cup	14%	.22	1.05	310.00	96.00	15.00
pepper, red, raw, ½ cup	10%	.25	2.50	3340.00	153.00	23.50
potato, baked, 1 medium	1%	.20	4.40	1.00	31.00	145.00
pumpkin, canned, 1 cup	8%	.70	4.50	15,680.00	12.00	80.00
rutabaga, cooked, 1 cup cubed*	3%	.20	4.80	940.00	36.00	60.00
spinach, fresh, 1 cup	11%	.18	3.90	4460.00	28.00	14.30
spinach, cooked, 1 cup	11%	.50	11.30	14,580	50.00	40.00
squash, acorn, cooked, 1 cup	8%	.29	4.01	1049.00	26.40	29.00
squash, butternut, cooked, 1 cup	1%	.18	2.60	16,800.00	36.20	83.00
squash, hubbard, cooked, 1 cup	9%	1.27	3.60	14,243.00	22.40	103.00
squash, spaghetti, cooked, 1 cup	6%	.40	2.20	171.00	5.50	45.00
squash, summer, cooked, 1 cup	6%	.20	5.80	820.00	21.00	29.00
squash, winter, cooked, 1 cup	7%	.70	6.76	9360.00	19.00	91.00
sweet potato, baked, 1 whole	4%	.70	4.10	24,877.00	25.00	160.00
sweet potatoes, canned, mashed 4 oz.	2%	.23	2.83	20,355.00	17.00	128.00
tomato, red, 1 medium	7%	.20	2.02	1110.00	28.00	25.00
tomatoes, cooked, 1 cup	7%	.50	5.74	2410.00	58.00	63.00
tomato juice, canned, 1 cup	5%	.24	.49	1940.00	39.00	45.00
tomato paste, canned, ½ cup	4%	.50	1.40	4325.00	.64	108.00
tomato sauce, canned, 1 cup	9%	.80	1.80	2660	44.00	78.00
turnip, raw, 1 cup diced	9%	.32	4.22	—	40.00	32.50
turnip, cooked, 1 cup diced	10%	.38	4.10	1.00	34.00	35.00
turnip greens, cooked, 1 cup	9%	.30	5.60	8270.00	68.00	30.00
watercress, chopped, ½ cup	14%	.03	.29	398.00	6.35	1.71
yams, cooked, 1 cup	1%	.20	7.80	24.00	10.00	238.00

BAKERY AND GRAIN PRODUCTS
Breads

	Cal from Fat	Grams Fat	Grams Fiber	IU Vit. A	Mg Vit. C	Cal
bagel, 1 whole	5%	1.00	.62	.10	—	165.00
corn bread, 1 serving, from mix	29%	4.20	4.00	100.00	—	130.00

cracked-wheat bread, 1 slice	8%	.60	1.45	1.00	— 66.00
French bread, 1 slice	10%	1.10	.07	1.00	— 102.00
Italian bread, 1 slice	2%	.20	.06	—	— 83.00
pita bread, 1 round	5%	1.20	1.00	—	— 198.00
raisin bread, 1 slice	10%	.70	.20	1.00	— 66.00
rye bread, 1 slice	4%	.30	1.01	—	— 61.00
pumpernickel, dark, 1 slice	5%	.40	2.00	—	— 79.00
white bread, soft, 1 slice	11%	.90	.70	1.00	— 75.00
whole wheat bread, soft, 1 slice	10%	.70	1.40	1.00	— 65.00

Cereals

All Bran, ⅓ cup	6%	.50	7.50	1231.00	14.70 70.00
Farina, cooked, 1 cup enriched	2%	.20	.60	—	— 116.00
rolled oats, cooked, 1 cup	15%	2.40	2.50	38.00	— 145.00
shredded wheat, 1 biscuit	3%	1.00	2.15	—	— 90.00
Wheatena, cooked, 1 cup	7%	1.10	3.30	—	— 135.00

Crackers

graham crackers, 4	21%	2.60	2.80	—	— 110.00
whole wheat crackers, 4	31%	2.20	1.20	—	— 64.00

Muffins and Misc.

bran muffin, 1	33%	3.90	1.50	90.00	— 105.00
cornmeal muffin, 1, from mix	29%	4.20	4.00	100.00	— 130.00
pasta, white, cooked, 1 cup	4%	.70	.56	—	— 172.00
pasta, whole wheat, 1 cup	4%	.70	4.94	—	— 172.00
plain muffin, 1	31%	4.00	.40	40.00	.13 118.00
popcorn, popped, plain, 1 cup	12%	.30	1.40	8.00	— 23.00
taco shell, 1	41%	2.20	.70	5.00	— 48.00
tortilla, corn, 1	43%	3.00	1.90	6.00	— 63.00
tortilla, flour, 1	17%	1.80	.60	2.00	— 95.00

GRAINS AND FLOURS

	Cal from Fat	Grams Fat	Grams Fiber	IU Vit. A	Mg Vit. C	Cal
barley, whole, cooked, ½ cup	7%	.80	2.30	—	—	100.00
bran, corn, 1 ounce	—	—	18.53	—	—	—
bran, oat, 1 ounce	—	—	7.88	—	—	—
bran, rice, 1 ounce	40%	5.48	3.26	—	—	78.80
bran, rye, 1 ounce	—	—	7.09	—	—	—
bran, wheat, 1 ounce	12%	1.30	11.22	—	—	60.30
brown rice, cooked, 1 cup	6%	1.56	4.50	—	—	232.00
bulgur wheat, cooked, 1 cup	3%	.90	7.10	—	—	246.00
buckwheat flour, 1 cup	7%	2.50	8.00	—	—	338.00
cake flour, enriched, 1 cup	3%	1.10	3.30	—	—	397.00
cornmeal, bolted, cooked, 1 cup	8%	4.15	11.00	590.00	—	442.00

dark rye flour, 1 cup	17%	5.90	12.00	70.00	— 313.00
millet, cooked, ½ cup	8%	.50	1.30	—	— 54.00
oats, rolled, dry, 1 cup	15%	5.10	5.70	82.00	— 311.00
soy flour, low-fat, 1 cup	17%	5.90	12.00	70.00	— 313.00
wheat flour, enriched, unbleached, 1 cup	2%	1.00	3.75	—	— 455.00
wheat germ, toasted, ¼ cup	27%	2.04	.50	—	— 68.00
white rice, cooked, 1 cup	2%	.51	1.64	—	— 237.00
whole wheat flour, 1 cup	5%	2.00	11.50	—	— 400.00
wild rice, cooked, ½ cup	2%	.20	2.56	—	— 92.00

DAIRY PRODUCTS
Cheese

	Cal from Fat	Grams Fat	Grams Fiber	IU Vit. A	Mg Vit. C	Cal
American, 1 ounce	72%	8.52	—	343.00	—	106.00
blue, 1 ounce	72%	8.00	—	204.00	—	100.00
Brie, 1 ounce	74%	7.80	—	189.00	—	95.00
cheddar, 1 ounce	73%	9.20	—	300.00	—	114.00
Colby, 1 ounce	71%	8.80	—	293.00	—	112.00
cottage cheese, creamed, 1 cup	37%	8.90	—	342.00	—	217.00
cottage cheese, 2% low-fat, 1 cup	19%	4.40	—	158.00	—	203.00
feta, 1 ounce	74%	6.20	—	325.00	—	75.00
Gouda, 1 ounce	69%	7.70	—	183.00	—	101.00
Gruyère, 1 ounce	70%	9.10	—	346.00	—	117.00
Monterey Jack, 1 ounce	71%	8.40	—	269.00	—	106.00
mozzarella, part-skim, 1 ounce	58%	4.60	—	166.00	—	72.00
mozzarella, whole milk, 1 ounce	65%	5.76	—	225.00	—	80.00
Parmesan, grated, ¼ cup	59%	6.10	—	142.00	—	92.00
ricotta, part-skim, 1 cup	50%	19.00	—	1063.00	—	340.00
ricotta, whole milk, 1 cup	67%	32.00	—	1205.00	—	428.00

Eggs

egg, whole, 1, hard cooked	64%	5.60	—	260.00	—	79.00
egg yolk, 1	80%	5.60	—	313.00	—	63.00

Ice Cream Products (Vanilla Flavor)

ice cream, regular, 1 cup	52%	15.40	—	543.00	.70	269.00
ice cream, rich, 1 cup	61%	23.70	—	897.00	.60	349.00
ice cream, soft-serve, 1 cup	61%	23.70	—	897.00	.60	349.00
ice milk, regular, 1 cup	28%	5.60	—	214.00	.80	184.00
ice milk, soft-serve, 1 cup	19%	4.60	—	175.00	1.20	223.00

Milk Products

buttermilk, 1 cup	20%	2.20	—	81.00	2.40	99.00

	Cal from Fat	Grams Fat	Grams Fiber	IU Vit. A	Mg Vit. C	Cal
cream, half-and-half, ¼ cup	63%	7.50	—	240.00	—	107.00
evaporated skim milk, ½ cup	2%	.30	—	500.00	1.60	99.00
evaporated whole milk, ½ cup	52%	9.80	—	306.00	2.40	169.00
instant nonfat dry milk, ⅓ cup	2%	.20	—	532.00	1.20	80.50
low-fat milk, 1%, 1 cup	22%	2.50	—	500.00	2.40	102.00
low-fat milk, 2%, 1 cup	36%	4.80	—	500.00	2.30	121.00
nonfat milk (skim), 1 cup	5%	.44	—	500.00	2.30	86.00
sour cream, ¼ cup	83%	11.30	—	454.00	.50	123.00
soy milk, fortified, 1 cup	51%	9.00	—	500.00	15.00	160.00
whipping cream, ¼ cup whipped	98%	11.10	—	437.00	.20	103.00
whole milk, 1 cup	49%	8.20	—	307.00	2.30	150.00
yogurt, plain, low-fat, 1 cup	22%	3.45	—	150.00	1.80	144.00

FISH, POULTRY, MEAT

Fish

	Cal from Fat	Grams Fat	Grams Fiber	IU Vit. A	Mg Vit. C	Cal
abalone, raw, 4 ounces	10%	1.20	—	—	—	112.00
bass, raw, 4 ounces	21%	2.60	—	1.14	—	114.00
bluefish, baked, 4 ounces	29%	5.90	—	57.10	—	182.00
catfish, raw, 4 ounces	19%	2.40	—	1.14	—	118.00
clams, raw, 4 ounces	17%	1.60	—	120.00	—	87.00
cod, steamed, 4 ounces	10%	1.02	—	1.14	—	95.00
crab, fresh, cooked, 4 ounces	12%	1.24	—	2461.00	2.30	96.00
crab, canned, 4 ounces	13%	1.90	—	34.00	.90	129.00
crawfish, raw, 4 ounces	14%	1.20	—	1.14	—	82.00
flounder, steamed, 4 ounces	18%	2.20	—	1.14	—	106.00
haddock, steamed, 4 ounces	7%	.90	—	57.00	—	112.00
halibut, steamed, 4 ounces	27%	4.60	—	91.00	—	150.00
lobster, boiled, 4 ounces	26%	3.90	—	1.14	—	136.00
mussels, raw, 4 ounces	20%	1.80	—	206.00	—	81.00
ocean perch, raw, 4 ounces	18%	2.30	—	34.00	3.40	113.00
octopus, raw, 4 ounces	10%	.90	—	1.14	—	83.40
oysters, raw, 4 ounces	25%	2.50	—	340.00	—	89.50
pike, raw, 4 ounces	9%	1.02	—	1.14	—	101.00
pollack, cooked, 4 ounces	1%	.07	—	1.14	—	113.00
prawns, cooked, 4 ounces	13%	1.70	—	1.14	—	122.00
salmon, steamed, 4 ounces	59%	14.80	—	183.00	—	225.00
salmon, pink, canned, 4 ounces	39%	6.70	—	80.00	—	154.00
sardines, canned in oil, drained, 4 ounces	52%	14.00	—	251.00	—	241.00
scallops, steamed 4 ounces	13%	1.71	—	—	.90	123.00
shrimp, cooked, 4 ounces	18%	2.70	—	1.14	—	134.00
snapper, baked, 4 ounces	11%	1.50	—	46.00	—	123.00
squid, raw, 4 ounces	16%	1.70	—	—	—	98.50
swordfish, raw, 4 ounces	33%	4.60	—	1806.00	—	125.00
trout, freshwater, fried, 4 ounces	51%	12.80	—	365.00	1.14	224.00
tuna, canned in water, 4 ounces	6%	.90	—	1.14	—	145.00

tuna, canned in oil, drained, 4 ounces	37%	9.40	—	91.40	— 225.00
tuna, raw, 4 ounces	31%	5.20	—	86.00	— 152.00

Poultry

chicken breast, with skin, roasted, 4 ounces	36%	8.82	—	105.00	— 223.00
chicken breast, meat only, 4 ounces	19%	4.04	—	23.80	— 187.00
chicken leg, with skin, roasted, 4 ounces	53%	15.30	—	153.00	— 263.00
chicken leg, meat only, roasted, 4 ounces	40%	9.50	—	71.00	— 216.00
duck, with skin, roasted, 4 ounces	76%	32.00	—	239.00	— 382.00
duck, meat only, roasted, 4 ounces	50%	12.70	—	88.00	— 228.00
goose, with skin, roasted, 4 ounces	65%	24.90	—	79.00	— 346.00
goose, meat only, roasted, 4 ounces	48%	14.30	—	—	— 270.00
turkey, light meat, meat only, roasted, 4 ounces	18%	3.60	—	—	— 177.00
turkey, dark meat, meat only, roasted, 4 ounces	35%	8.20	—	—	— 212.00

Beef

beef liver, cooked, 3 ounces	45%	9.80	—	21,613.00	23.00 195.00
beef tongue, cooked, 3 ounces	62%	15.80	—	—	1.70 230.00
ground beef, 10% fat, cooked, 3 ounces	47%	9.60	—	20.00	— 185.00
ground beef, 21% fat, cooked, 3 ounces	68%	18.40	—	31.00	— 244.00
pot roast, lean, with some fat, 3 ounces	73%	20.00	—	30.00	— 246.00
pot roast, lean only, 3 ounces	41%	7.40	—	10.00	— 164.00
rib roast, lean, with some fat, 3 ounces	81%	33.50	—	70.00	— 374.00
rib roast, lean only, 3 ounces	50%	11.40	—	20.00	— 205.00
round steak, lean, with some fat, 3 ounces	52%	12.80	—	20.00	— 222.00
round steak, lean only, 3 ounces	30%	5.30	—	10.00	— 161.00
rump roast, lean, with some fat, 3 ounces	72%	21.50	—	40.00	— 269.00
rump roast, lean only, 3 ounces	44%	7.90	—	10.00	— 162.00
sirloin steak, lean, with some fat, 3 ounces	89%	32.60	—	50.00	— 329.00
sirloin steak, lean only, 3 ounces	31%	6.10	—	15.10	— 175.00

Lamb

lamb chop, lean, with some fat, 3 ounces	76%	27.50	—	1.00	—	325.00
lamb chop, lean only, 3 ounces	48%	9.70	—	1.50	—	184.00
leg of lamb, lean, with some fat, 3 ounces	61%	15.70	—	—	—	232.00
leg of lamb, lean only, 3 ounces	37%	6.50	—	1.00	—	160.00
shoulder roast, lean, with some fat, 3 ounces	73%	22.70	—	—	—	278.00
shoulder roast, lean only, 3 ounces	48%	9.00	—	—	—	170.00

Pork

loin roast, lean, with some fat, 3 ounces	71%	24.20	—	—	—	308.00
loin roast, lean only, 3 ounces	50%	12.10	—	—	—	216.00
loin chop, lean, with some fat, 3 ounces	70%	23.70	—	—	—	307.00
loin chop, lean only, 3 ounces	52%	12.20	—	—	—	211.00
shoulder, lean, with some fat, 3 ounces	83%	27.80	—	—	—	300.00
shoulder, lean only, 3 ounces	72%	16.60	—	—	—	207.00
spare ribs, 3 ounces edible portion	84%	33.30	—	—	—	359.00

Cured Pork and Pork Products

bacon, regular, cooked, 3 slices	77%	9.40	—	—	6.40	109.00
bologna, beef, 1 slice	81%	6.52	—	—	4.00	72.00
bologna, turkey, 1 slice	69%	4.30	—	—	—	56.50
breakfast sausage, 1 link	76%	4.05	—	—	—	48.00
breakfast sausage, 1 patty	76%	8.40	—	—	.50	100.00
Canadian bacon, cooked, 1 slice	41%	2.00	—	—	5.00	43.00
frankfurter, beef, 1	82%	16.80	—	—	14.00	184.00
frankfurter, turkey, 1	73%	8.30	—	—	—	102.00
ham, extra lean, sliced lunchmeat, 3 ounces	34%	4.30	—	—	21.20	112.00
ham, regular, with some fat, roasted, 3 ounces	67%	14.20	—	—	—	207.00
ham, lean only, roasted, 3 ounces	32%	4.70	—	—	—	133.00
Italian sausage, 1 link	72%	17.20	—	—	1.00	216.00
knockwurst, 1 link	81%	18.90	—	—	18.00	209.00
liver pate, canned, 1 ounce	80%	7.90	—	936.00	—	89.40
liverwurst, 1 ounce	78%	8.10	—	—	—	93.00
pepperoni, 1 ounce	81%	12.40	—	—	—	139.00
salami, beef, 1 ounce	72%	5.70	—	—	3.70	71.40

Veal

veal cutlet, 3 ounces	46%	9.40	—	—	— 184.00
veal rib roast, no bones, 3 ounces	51%	12.10	—	—	— 212.00

SEEDS AND NUTS

	Cal from Fat	Grams Fat	Grams Fiber	IU Vit. A	Mg Vit. C	Cal
almonds, whole, roasted, ¼ cup	83%	22.60	5.60	—	—	246.00
brazil nuts, 10	92%	27.10	3.60	4.28	—	264.00
cashews, roasted, ¼ cup	73%	15.90	2.12	35.00	—	196.00
chestnuts, dry, 1 ounce	10%	1.20	1.90	—	—	108.00
coconut, fresh, grated, ¼ cup	91%	7.05	2.70	—	—	69.70
macadamia nuts, ¼ cup	99%	25.20	2.03	—	—	230.00
peanut butter, ¼ cup	78%	33.50	5.00	—	—	386.00
peanuts, roasted, ¼ cup	77%	18.00	2.90	9.50	—	210.00
pecans, chopped, ¼ cup	93%	21.00	1.80	37.50	.50	203.00
pine nuts, 1 ounce	71%	13.40	.25	4.00	—	170.00
pistachio nuts, ¼ cup	81%	18.80	1.75	81.20	—	210.00
poppy seeds, ¼ cup	75%	15.70	2.20	—	—	188.00
pumpkin/squash seeds, dry, ¼ cup	76%	16.30	.67	25.00	—	194.00
sesame seeds, whole ¼ cup	78%	18.40	2.40	11.20	—	211.00
sunflower seeds, dry, ¼ cup	76%	17.10	1.37	17.50	—	203.00
tahini (sesame butter), ¼ cup	80%	48.00	2.00	—	—	540.00
walnuts, chopped, ¼ cup	85%	18.60	1.55	95.00	—	196.00

FATS AND OILS

	Cal from Fat	Grams Fat	Grams Fiber	IU Vit. A	Mg Vit. C	Cal
butter, 1 tablespoon	100%	11.50	—	434.00	—	102.00
lard, 1 tablespoon	100%	12.90	—	—	—	115.50
liquid oil (such as corn), 1 tablespoon	100%	13.50	—	—	—	120.30
margarine, 1 tablespoon	100%	11.40	—	469.00	—	102.00

CONDIMENTS AND SPREADS

	Cal from Fat	Grams Fat	Grams Fiber	IU Vit. A	Mg Vit. C	Cal
barbeque sauce, 1 tablespoon	68%	1.10	.10	56.20	.80	14.20
catsup, 1 tablespoon	3%	.07	.08	239.00	2.50	18.10
horseradish, prepared, 1 tablespoon	0%	—	.14	—	.60	6.00

mayonnaise, 1 tablespoon	100%	10.90	—	38.70	—	98.50
mayonnaise-type dressing, 1 tablespoon	77%	4.90	—	32.30	—	57.20
mayonnaise-type dressing, low-calorie, 1 tablespoon	75%	2.90	—	34.30	—	34.70
mustard, prepared, 1 tablespoon	53%	.69	—	1.50	—	11.70
olives, green, pitted, 4	100%	2.00	.69	48.00	—	18.00
olives, black, pitted, 4	100%	3.80	.83	20.80	—	31.20
pickle, dill, 1	13%	.10	.33	70.00	4.00	7.00
pickle, sweet, 1	2%	.04	.08	10.00	1.00	22.00
tarter sauce, 1 tablespoon	99%	8.10	.04	30.00	—	74.00

SAUCES

	Cal from Fat	Grams Fat	Grams Fiber	IU Vit. A	Mg Vit. C	Cal
béarnaise sauce, ¼ cup	100%	24.40	.05	981.00	1.75	221.00
bordelaise sauce, ¼ cup	76%	6.50	.20	33.00	.40	77.00
cheese sauce, ¼ cup	68%	7.70	.08	340.00	.30	102.00
chocolate sauce, thin, 1 tablespoon	5%	.24	.47	3.75	—	48.70
cranberry sauce, canned, 1 tablespoon	1%	.03	.48	3.40	.34	26.10
hollandaise sauce, ¼ cup	100%	24.40	—	946.00	1.22	220.00
Mornay sauce, ¼ cup	73%	12.80	—	540.00	.40	159.00
tomato sauce, ½ cup	9%	.40	1.00	1330.00	22.00	39.00
white sauce, ½ cup	65%	6.90	.12	360.00	.48	95.50

SWEETENERS

	Cal from Fat	Grams Fat	Grams Fiber	IU Vit. A	Mg Vit. C	Cal
apple butter, 1 tablespoon	4%	.14	.20	—	.04	33.00
corn syrup, light 1 tablespoon	—	—	—	—	—	59.40
corn syrup, dark, 1 tablespoon	—	—	—	—	—	59.40
honey, 1 tablespoon	—	—	—	—	—	64.40
jams/preserves, 1 tablespoon	—	.02	.12	2.00	—	54.00
jellies, 1 tablespoon	—	.02	—	2.00	.70	49.00
maple syrup, 1 tablespoon	—	—	—	—	—	50.00
marmalade, 1 tablespoon	—	—	—	—	—	52.00
molasses, blackstrap, 1 tablespoon	—	—	—	—	—	50.00
pancake syrup, 1 tablespoon	—	—	—	—	—	51.00
sugar, brown, 1 tablespoon	—	—	—	—	—	51.30
sugar, white, 1 tablespoon	—	—	—	—	—	48.90
sugar, powdered, 1 tablespoon	—	—	—	—	—	28.86

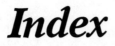

Index